ATHEROSCLEROTIC CARDIOVASCULAR DISEASE

Edited by **Ksenija Pešek**

Atherosclerotic Cardiovascular Disease
Edited by Ksenija Pešek

Published by InTech

Janeza Trdine 9, 51000 Rijeka, Croatia

Publishing Process Manager Romina Krebel

Technical Editor Teodora Smiljanic

Cover Designer InTech Design Team

Additional hard copies can be obtained from orders@intechopen.com

Atherosclerotic Cardiovascular Disease, Edited by Ksenija Pešek
p. cm.
ISBN 978-953-307-695-9

For EU product safety concerns:
IN TECH d.o.o., Prolaz Marije Krucifikse Kozulić 3, 51000 Rijeka, Croatia,
info@intechopen.com or visit our website at intechopen.com.

Meet the editor

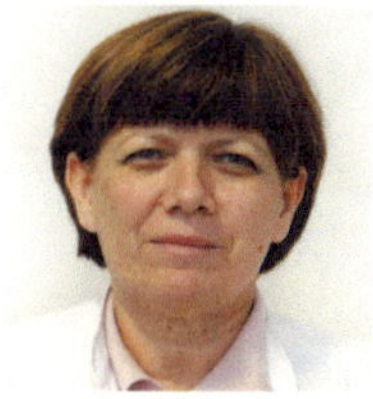

Ksenija Pešek, MD. has been employed in the capacity of Specialist Internist at the Cardiology Department of the Zabok General Hospital since 1992. As the Head of the Cardiology Department, she has been the chief mentor to resident doctors and resident cardiology specialists at the hospital. She is a regular lecturer in Cardiology at the Department of Internal Medicine at the Zabok General Hospital, as well as the rest of the county. In 2008 she has been awarded the title of Primarius and Cardiologist. Since 2008 she has been active as Vice President of the Croatian Cardiology Society. She is also a member of the European Cardiology Association, of the Croatian Association for Hypertension, and the Croatian Internist Association. She has participated in all the leading clinical studies in the field of cardiology in Croatia and has published 15 professional and scientific works in cardiology. With her long career and professional and scientific works in cardiology, she has contributed significantly to the science, and has as well excelled in the clinical, educational and organizational aspect of cardiology. Since 2010 she has been an active member of FESC (Fellow of European society of Cardiology).

Contents

Preface

Cardiovascular diseases (CVD) are still one of the leading causes of death in the world. This book is another contribution to the application of new knowledge in the area of CVD. Authors of this book are from different parts of the world and of different cultures.

Over the past 20 years, numerous epidemiological, basic, laboratory and clinical tests have been conducted in the area of cardiology. Epidemiological studies confirmed the strong association between risk factors for coronary disease, gene disorders that could cause cardiac disease were discovered, recent studies of new methods in the treatment of CVD and their prevention, as well as the prevention of cardiac death were conducted.

Medical books are a set of facts which with each new reading give a different view of the observed changes. Small changes are important. Medicine is changing slowly but constantly. Same is with all new editions of books on medicine; the book is getting better every time and provides more. A series of small changes in all aspects of medicine leads to significant changes. To understand these changes, they should be constantly monitored.

Our task is to enable that knowledge and new information from this field become instantly available to a wider range of doctors and other medical professionals. I hope this book will provide greater visibility and access to detection and treatment of vulnerable patients.

I wish to express my gratitude to everyone for their effort and time, helping with valuable facts and opinions, thus making possible for this book to be published. Colleagues, using this edition, we meet the requirements of our responsible and hard, but human calling.

Ksenija Pešek, MD, FESC
Cardiology Clinic Zabok
Croatia

Part 1

General Considerations of Cardiovascular Disease

1

The Importance of Risk Factors Analysis in the Prevention of Cardiovascular Disease (CVD)

Ksenija Pešek, Tomislav Pešek and Siniša Roginić
Cardiology Clinic Zabok
Croatia

1. Introduction

1.1 Cardiovascular disease

Cardiovascular diseases (CVD) are the number one killer of modern humankind. According to the World Health Organization (WHO) about 17.5 million people die every year from cardiovascular diseases and it is estimated this number will increase up to 20 million by 2015. Although genetic factors have a significant impact on the cardiovascular disease occurrence, their importance is often overestimated. The results of numerous clinical and epidemiological studies emphasise that cardiovascular diseases can often be predicted and therefore preventable. Accordingly, it is possible to discern several important, independent disease risk factors wich can be affected to a greater or less extent.

1.1.1 Definition

Cardiovascular diseases are caused by arterial lesions characterized by local intimae thickening consisting of proliferating, altered smooth muscle cells, macrophages, lipids from intracellular and extracellular serum lipoprotein deposits and proliferating connective tissue (collagen, elastin, mucopolysaccharides. Consequential arterial narrowing causes CVD, stroke, and peripheral arterial disease. The risk factors leading to the development and occurrence of cardiovascular disease are arterial hypertension, cigarette smoking, hypercholesterolemia, hypertriglyceridemia, diabetes mellitus and positive family history. Additional factors favouring the occurrence of cardiovascular disease include obesity, sedentary lifestyle (insufficient physical activity) and emotional stress. Cardiovascular diseases are associated with high morbidity and mortality rates, thus posing a major health and socioeconomic problem to modern society. CVD are the world's the leading cause of death and severe disability. CVD or ischemic heart disease occur due to reduction of coronary blood flow, most commonly caused by coronary thrombus. This results in myocardial lesions, whose extent determine the symptomatology, clinical course and disease outcome. According to symptomatology and clinical course, ischemic heart disease is categorized into acute coronary syndrome (ST-segment elevation myocardial infarction - STEMI, non-ST-segment elevation myocardial infarction – NSTEMI and unstable angina) and stable angina pectoris. In almost 99% of cases, CVD are caused by obstructive atherosclerosis and less frequently by spasm (usually idiopathic, or caused by drugs such as cocaine). Subintimal plaques reducing or obstructing coronary blood flow characterize atherosclerosis.

Strict prevention of risk factors in patients with established CVD and those with high-risk profile can reduce the incidence and recurrence of clinical complications - coronary artery disease, stroke and peripheral arterial disease. It is crucial to focus on the prevention of disability and premature death. Coronary atherosclerosis typically develops insidiously; it is irregularly distributed through vascular bed. Acute coronary syndrome occurs due to sudden obstruction of blood flow to heart muscle, mainly due to rupture of eccentric atherosclerotic plaque. Major clinical presentations of coronary heart disease are stable angina pectoris, unstable angina and myocardial infarction. Risk factors include high levels of LDL-cholesterol, low HDL-cholesterol level, high triglyceride level, smoking, diet and lifestyle as well as systemic diseases like arterial hypertension and diabetes. The association between serum total cholesterol and LDL-cholesterol levels with risk of coronary heart disease is now well recognized and enduring. HDL-cholesterol is inversely associated with risk of coronary heart disease. Reduction of serum LDL-cholesterol slows the progression of coronary heart disease. Reduced LDL-cholesterol was also beneficial in those patients with existing coronary heart disease even if their LDL-cholesterol is within normal limits.

1.1.2 The risk factors

Division of CVD risk factors into modifiable and non-modifiable is very useful because it shows us where to direct our efforts in cardiovascular prevention. Major modifiable risk factors are: high levels of total and LDL cholesterol, low HDL-cholesterol levels, high triglyceride levels, high blood pressure, diabetes (or glucose intolerance), cigarette smoking, obesity, insufficient consumption of fruits and vegetables, lack of regular exercise, personality structure and stressful social environment.

Unfortunately, we cannot affect cardiovascular risk derived from family history, age and sex.

Risk factors mentioned above insidiously lead to development and occurrence of cardiovascular diseases. Hypercholesterolemia, one of the major modifiable risk factor is important in symptomatic and in asymptomatic patients. It is important to analyze total cholesterol and also its main lipoprotein particles (LDL and HDL cholesterol) which are also parameters of increased CVD risk.

1.2 Atherosclerosis

Atherosclerosis is pathological process characterized by formation of subintimal plaques that can reduce or obstruct blood flow through the vessel. It is a result of normal blood vessels ageing, with initial lesion developing before age 30 (so-called fatty streaks). Risk factors that significantly accelerate this process are serum lipid impairment, hypertension, cigarette smoking, diabetes mellitus, obesity, physical inactivity and hereditary factors i.e. positive family history of cardiovascular disorders. Elevated level of low-density lipoprotein (LDL) and decreased level of high-density lipoprotein (HDL) strongly predispose the development of atherosclerosis. As mentioned above, so-called protective HDL-cholesterol is inversely proportional to the risk of CVD. Main causes of its decrease are cigarette smoking, obesity and inadequate physical activity. Premenopausal women usually have higher HDL levels then men due to hormonal effects of estrogen and therefore lower incidence of CVD. This protective effect vanishes in postmenopause. The cholesterol level and the incidence of CVD are strongly influenced by environmental factors including diet.

Besides hyperlipoproteinemia, arterial hypertension is another major risk factor for the occurrence and progression of atherosclerotic lesions. The main pathophysiological

mechanism is mechanical damage to endothelial cells due to altered hemodynamics, i.e. enhanced force of the blood flow, or formation of whirls at vascular bifurcations.
Arteriosclerosis is a general term describing hardening (and loss of elasticity) of medium or large arteries. Atherosclerosis is arteriosclerosis caused by atheromatous plaque. Arteriolosclerosis is a narrowing of small arteries caused by its wall thickening. In recent years, development of atherosclerosis has been elucidated (figure 1).

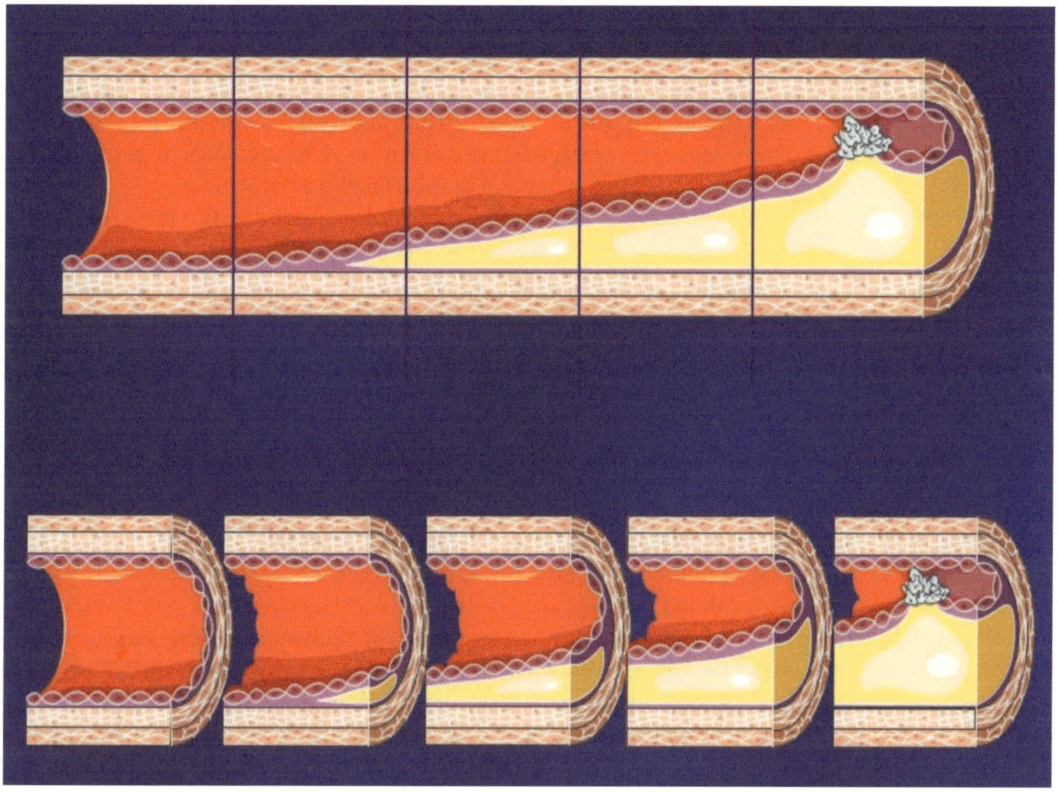

Fig. 1. Progression of atherosclerosis from fatty streak, formation of subintimal plaque, further lipid deposition and finally plaque rupture with subsequent thrombogenesis (Figure was produced using Servier Medical Art).

Atherosclerosis remains the major cause of death and premature disability in developed societies. It is predicted that by the year 2020. cardiovascular diseases (notably atherosclerosis) will become the leading global cause of total disease burden. Etiology of atherosclerosis is very complex, but outcome remains the same - reduction of blood flow through various organs leading to distinct clinical entities. Coronary atherosclerosis commonly causes myocardial infarction and angina pectoris. Atherosclerosis of the cerebral arteries frequently provokes strokes and transient cerebral ischemia. Atherosclerosis of the peripheral vessels causes intermittent claudicating, gangrene and mesenteric ischemia. Atherosclerosis can affect the kidneys either directly or as a frequent site of atheroembolism. Some regions are particularly susceptible to atheromatous lesions, respectively bifurcations. For example, proximal left anterior descending (LAD) coronary artery exhibits a particular predilection for developing atherosclerosis disease. Likewise, atherosclerosis preferentially affects the proximal portions of the renal arteries and carotid bifurcation, in the extracranial brain circulation. Not all manifestations of atherosclerosis result from stenotic, occlusive disease. Ecstasies and development of aneurismal disease (pathological widening of blood vessel), for example, frequently occur in the aorta. In addition to local, flow-limiting stenoses, non-occlusive intimal atherosclerosis also occur diffusely in affected arteries, as shown by intravascular ultrasound and postmortem studies.

Atherogenesis in human typically occurs gradually over a period of many decades. Atherosclerotic plaques growth probably does not occur in a smooth, linear fashion, but rather discontinuously, with periods of relative quiescence punctuated by periods of rapid progression. After a prolonged silent period, atherosclerosis may clinically manifest itself in acute or chronic fashion (stable angina, reproducible intermittent claudicating or acute coronary syndrome). Some people never experience clinical manifestation of arterial disease despite the presence of widespread atherosclerosis demonstrated post-mortem.

The endothelial monolayer overlying the intimae contacts blood. Its' structural and functional consistency is the first dam for development of atherosclerosis. Hypercholesterolemia promotes accumulation of LDL-particles in the intimae. The lipoprotein particles then associate with constituents of the extracellular matrix, notably proteolytic enzymes. Sequestration within the intimae separates lipoproteins from some plasma antioxidants and favours oxidative modification. Such modified lipoprotein particles may trigger a local inflammatory response responsible for signaling subsequent steps in lesion formation. The augmented expression of various leukocytes adhesion molecules recruits monocytes to the site of a nascent arterial lesion.

Once adherent, some white blood cells will migrate to the intimae attracted by the factors including modified lipoprotein particles themselves and chemo attractant cytokines, such as the chemokine macrophage chemo attractant protein-1 produced by vascular wall cells in response to modified lipoproteins. Leukocytes in the evolving fatty streak can divide and exhibit augmented expression of receptors for modified lipoproteins. These mononuclear phagocytes ingest lipids and become foam cells, represented by a cytoplasm filled with lipid droplets. As the fatty streak evolves into a more complicated atherosclerotic lesion, smooth-muscle cells migrate through the internal elastic membrane and accumulate within the expanding intimae where they lay down extracellular matrix that forms the bulk of the advanced lesion. Depending on the lipid compound, plaques are divided into stable and unstable. Stable plaques contain smaller amount of ingested lipids covered with thick fibrous layer thus preventing its rupture. On the other hand, unstable plaques with high lipid content and thin fibrous cap are very vulnerable and their rupture initiates acute ischemic event.

2. Modifiable risk factors

2.1 Blood pressure (BP)

High blood pressure is the arterial pressure of above normal limits (traditionally 140/90 mmHg). It is commonly called the silent killer because it damages vital organs (brain, heart, kidneys) without causing any early symptoms. Untreated hypertension increases the risk of heart failure, heart attack (myocardial infarction), stroke, aneurysms, kidney failure and damage to retinal blood vessels. Hypertension is marked by rise in blood pressure regardless of the cause, and is divided into primary (essential) and secondary hypertension. In most (95%) cases etiology is multifactorial and incompletely understood and this is called primary or essential hypertension. Secondary hypertension (5%) results from damage of organs involved in regulation of blood pressure, endocrine disorders and drug toxicity. Children and adolescents have significantly lower blood pressure than adults do. Blood pressure naturally exhibits diurnal variation. Physiologically blood pressure varies throughout day with the highest values in the morning and lowest during sleep at night. Arterial blood pressure usually progressively increases with age because great arteries lose their natural elasticity and become rigid. There are two basic mechanisms of increased blood pressure - vasoconstriction (contraction of the arteries) usually caused by hormones or stress and the increase in total blood circulating volume. Obesity, sedentary lifestyle, stress, excessive alcohol and fatty foods intake have an important role in hypertension. These causes are potentially modifiable and by doing so hypertension can be avoided unless, there is a hereditary, constitutional cause of hypertension. Stress temporary increases blood pressure by activating biochemical processes that cause vasoconstriction of blood vessels. This can partly explain the mechanism of hypertension.

A diagnosis of arterial hypertension and all treatment decisions rely on the correct measurement of arterial blood pressure. The clinical measurement of arterial pressure using a calibrated mercury sphygmomanometer is still the main method in everyday clinical practice but it demands compliance with certain rules and recommendations. Because of the latest knowledge, and particularly chronobiology, we are increasingly aware of this method's limitations, primarily due to the characteristics of the measurement variable itself. A more comprehensive picture from arterial pressure (AP) values can be obtained by an intermittent 24-hour measurement of arterial pressure, and mean values obtained with this method are the closest to real values. Self-measurement of the arterial pressure cannot fully replace the intermittent arterial pressure measurement, but it can represent an additional source of information in diagnostic procedures and treatment decisions. Patient education and certified sphyngomanometers are mandatory to avoid false positive and negative measurements. Both intermittent AP measurement and self-measurement have shown to be superior in the prediction of target organ damage and its progression to clinical measurement. When applying these methods, it is important to use devices authorized by international professional societies. The appropriate combination of more measurement methods is the only proper way to make an accurate diagnosis of arterial hypertension, asses total cardiovascular risk, and make the safest decision on treatment method.

Arterial hypertension is an important risk factor for both cardiovascular and renal disease. Blood pressure control is important to prevent complications that may attribute to elevated blood pressure.

Treatment of arterial hypertension is base on two important principles: application of non-pharmacological measures or lifestyle changes, and pharmacotherapy. The new ESH/ESC (European Society of Hypertension/European Society of Cardiology) guidelines for arterial hypertension diagnosis and treatment emphasize the importance of total cardiovascular risk assessment in addition to blood pressure values. This means that a person with normal mean blood pressure can have higher cardiovascular risk then hypertensive person without additional risk factors. New laboratory tests and diagnostic procedures have been introduced in order to stratify cardiovascular risk of hypertensive patients. Routine assessment of target organ damage (especially heart, kidney and retina) now includes, among others, microalbuminuria and measurement or estimation of glomerular filtration rate.

Main treatment goals are reduction of target organ damage and prevention of cardiovascular events. Lifestyle changes are recommended to all patients and represent main stem of therapy in spite of wide spectrum of medications. The Guidelines have kept their educational and advisory character, emphasizing individual approach to patients, thus trying to improve implementation in everyday practice.

2.1.1 Isolated systolic hypertension

Introduction of isolated systolic hypertension as a separate entity confirmed the importance of systolic blood pressure as cardiovascular risk factors, indicating the need to treat this form of hypertension particularly prevalent in elderly and very elderly patients. It is defined as systolic blood pressure above 140 mmHg, with diastolic values below 90 mmHg.
The goal of therapy for more patients is BP under 140/90 mmHg, but for diabetic patients and individuals at high or very high total CVD risk, the BP threshold should be lower (130/80 mmHg). In patients with established CVD, the BP goal is < 130/85 mmHg and the choice of antihypertensive drugs depends on the underlying cardiovascular disease, concomitant disease, and the presence or absence of other cardiovascular risk factors. In asymptomatic individuals, the decision to start treatment depends on not only the level of BP, but also the assessment of total cardiovascular risk and the presence or absence of subclinical target organ damage. BP reduction should generally be obtained gradually.
Elevated BP, whether systolic or diastolic, is established as a strong, independent risk factor for renal disease and for several cardiovascular (CV) disorders-including coronary heart disease (CVD), stroke, heart failure and peripheral arterial disease.

2.1.2 Definition and classification of hypertension

From a prognostic point of view, there is no clear cut-off value do define hypertension because BP distribution in population follows Gaussian curve. This has major implications for definition of hypertension particularly since there is no distinctive BP level at which risk of CV or renal disorder starts. On the contrary, CV risk is continuous and graded across the whole BP range and hence from a prognostic viewpoint the definition of hypertension is arbitrary. Nevertheless, for practical and communication purposes hypertension is considered and defined as a separate entity, as if it were a dichotomous (present/absent) variable. The pragmatic determinant of the definition of hypertension should be that level of BP at which investigation and management do more good than harm as determined by randomizes clinical trial (RCT) evidence. In fact, evidence supporting current definition of hypertension most commonly used around the world is not based on RCT evidence but rather based on overall evidence. Nevertheless, the current definitions still seem reasonable. Whilst the definition of hypertension (systolic BP>140 mmHg and/or, diastolic BP 90>mmHg) is universally accepted for the classification of BP (Table 1 and 2).
The importance of raised BP lies in the fact that it is one of the major risk factors for current global mortality. Indeed raised BP, here defined as a systolic BP> 115 mmHg, is current the biggest single contributor to death around the world.
Prevalence of hypertension, defined as a systolic BP>140 mmHg and/or a diastolic BP >90 mmHg varies around the world. Hypertensions rates also vary with age and sex. BP tend to rise with age in both men and women once populations have become exposed to the adverse environmental factors associated with development of hypertension (i.e. advanced age, excess salt, calories, saturated fat and alcohol intakes with reduced intake of fresh fruit

Category	Systolic	Diastolic
Optimal	<120	<80
Normal	120 - 129	80 - 84
High normal	130 - 139	85 - 89
Grade 1 hypertension (mild)	140 - 159	90 - 99
Grade 2 hypertension (moderate)	160 - 179	100 - 109
Grade 3 hypertension (severe)	≥180	≥110
Isolated systolic hypertension	≥ 140	<90

Table 1. Classification of BP levels: European Guidelines

BP classification	Systolic BP (mmHg)	Diastolic BP (mmHg)
Normal	<120	<80
Prehypertension	120 - 139	80 - 89
Stage 1 hypertension	140 - 159	90 - 99
Stage 2 hypertension	≥ 160	≥110

Table 2. Classification of BP levels: American Guidelines

and vegetables and reduced exercise output). Until the age of 60, hypertension is usually more common in men than women but after then even higher rates are apparent among women. It is also clear than in many parts of the world including the established market economies, hypertension affects the majority of adults over the age of 60 years and presents a major public health issue.

By contrast, in several remote uncultivated populations around the world BP levels show the natural relationship between BP an increased age. These data taken from the Intersalt study showed no increase in systolic or diastolic BP across the age range 20 to 60 years in populations around the world that were not exposed to adverse environment factors.

Future prospects for the prevalence of hypertension: Because 80% of the world's population is in the process of development, humongous increase in hypertension prevalence is expected. It is therefore even more important that optimal BP management is determined and put into practice.

Why will the prevalence of hypertension increase? The absolute number of people affected by raised blood pressure will rise over the next 2 decades in part because the world population is increasing and the mean age of the world's population (accompanied by hypertension) is increasing. Paradoxically in developing communities, adverse changes first arise in people from the higher socio-economic strata (SES). Consequently, it is in this part of society that strokes and coronary events first tend to appear. As the development, process continues the exposure to risk factor reverses and the CVD are more prevalent in the lower SES.

Based on the large prospective observational data both systolic and diastolic BP show a strong direct relationship with all major adverse cardiovascular events, including coronary heart disease (CHD), stroke, cardiovascular mortality and heart failure.

Although the relationship varies by age and sex, a 20-mmHg rise in systolic BP or a 10-mmHg rise in diastolic BP doubles the cardiovascular (CV) risk. Support for this linear association between increased BP and risk of CV events arise from the results of hypertension treatment. Meta-analyses of these trial data consistently and clearly show that BP reduction is effective in reducing CV events. Highly significant and clinically important reductions of stroke and CHD events and vascular deaths were apparent using these agents. Interestingly the benefits in terms of CHD events reduction were less than those expected from prospective observational data. Nevertheless, 10-20 mmHg average reduction in BP achieved in the trials improves CHD prevention.

2.1.3 High blood pressure - hypertension

It is the one of most prevalent cardiovascular disorder, but is also a high-risk factor for the development of coronary heart disease. Compared with normal blood pressure in healthy subjects, hypertension increases the risk of developing CVD fivefold. In people over the age of 45, high blood pressure is the main risk factor for the development of myocardial infarction. However, the risk for development of myocardial infarction increases with blood pressure in all age groups. Treatment of hypertension results in clear reduction of associated disorders such a myocardial insufficiency, renal disorders and stroke. Those who are 65 years or more benefit most from a reduction of raised blood pressure in terms of prevention of myocardial infarction. Borderline hypertension in the young is an indicator of increased risk for cardiovascular disease in older age, therefore early prevention and prophylactic treatment is advised.

2.2 Lipids

Lipids are not water-soluble and their transport in blood is only possible in complexes with protein-apoprotein. Lipoprotein particles have spherical shape. Their main goal is the transfer of lipids and fat-soluble vitamins. They consist of hydrophobic core containing nonpolar lipids (triglycerides and esterified cholesterol) and hydrophilic surface layer of polar lipids (phospholipids and nonesterified cholesterol).

Apoproteins are located on the surface but their nonpolar part reaches the core particles. The main metabolic role of apoprotein is to act as a cofactor of some enzymes involved in the metabolism of lipoprotein particles and to bind to specific receptors on the surface of various cells and thus facilitate the entry of lipoproteins into them and catabolism of these particles in the cells. Lipoproteins are divided as follows:

1. Chylomicrons
2. Very low density lipoprotein - VLDL
3. Low density lipoprotein - LDL
4. High density lipoproteins - HDL
5. Intermediate density lipoproteins - IDL

The largest particles - chylomicrons transport triglycerides and cholesterol ingested in meals from the small intestine to the liver. Bloodstream is abundant with chylomicrons after meal, especially the one rich and fat. VLDL particles are synthesized in the liver and transport triglycerides and cholesterol to the heart muscle and adipose tissue. Since VLDL particles hydrolyze triglyceride and release smaller particles IDL particles during their travel through bloodstream, they are believed to promote atherosclerosis. LDL particles are the product of VLDL catabolism and mainly consist of cholesterol. LDL carries cholesterol from the liver and blood cells. Excess of cholesterol not used by cells is deposited in artery walls. Gradually, deposited cholesterol and other substances create plaque, which can eventually cause a blockage of blood vessel. HDL particles contain more protein than any other lipoprotein. HDL circulates through the blood and removes excess cholesterol from the blood and tissues, returning it to the liver from where one can again be incorporated into LDL. High HDL cholesterol levels are associated with low levels of chylomicrons, VLDL remnants, LDL and consequently a lower risk of atherosclerosis.

HDL-cholesterol particles are rich in cholesterol, but it is descended from the atherosclerotic fatty deposits on artery walls where it is in surplus. Therefore, the particles are protective, preventing the development of atherosclerosis.

Unlike HDL-cholesterol, LDL-cholesterol particles, which also has the highest cholesterol content are highly atherogenic and play a key role in various stages of atherosclerosis.

Increased amount of LDL-cholesterol in the blood is the most important etiological factor for the occurrence of coronary heart disease and myocardial infarction. Low HDL-cholesterol is also an important risk factor. Clinical importance of diagnosing and treating dyslipidemia is prevention of emergence and development of atherosclerosis and its major clinical forms - coronary heart disease and myocardial infarction.

Relation between level of cholesterol (especially LDL-cholesterol) and CVD risk is supported by data from studies of patients with a family hypercholesterolemia. Heterozygous for this disease usually die in the fifties of myocardial infarction, while homozygous have even higher cholesterol levels and die from CVD before age 20.

Epidemiological studies in different countries in the world, which include socio-economic conditions and diet, show a direct correlation between the concentration cholesterol in blood and mortality from CVD. There is no population with high CVD and overall low cholesterol level in the blood. In case of exceptions, there are other risk factors for CVD.

It is interesting to notice that the Japanese, who live in Japan on local diet with low concentration of cholesterol, after migrating to USA, acquire dietary habits of the host country and their level of blood cholesterol is much greater than in Japan. Consequently, the incidence of coronary disease is increased.

High triglycerides blood level is also a risk factor for cardiovascular disease, but less important than hypercholesterolemia.

In contrast to hypercholesterolemia, where CVD risk rises with concentration of cholesterol in the blood, the biggest risk arises with moderate increase in triglyceride level. Hypertriglyceridemia is regularly accompanied by a decreased HDL-cholesterol and low HDL-cholesterol is an important atherosclerotic risk factor, independent of other factors. VLDL and IDL particles, both rich in triglycerides have atherogenic effect and hypertriglyceridemia promotes thrombogenesis and inhibits fibrinolysis. Only extremely severe hypertriglyceridemia (greater than 10 mmol/L) increases risk of acute pancreatitis. Increase in levels of special types of lipoprotein particles Lipoprotein (a) (Lp (a)) which are similar in composition to LDL particles, but also containing Apo (a), (intervenes in the process of thrombogenesis), is an independent risk factor for atherosclerosis.

2.2.1 Dyslipidemia

Dyslipidemia is defined as an abnormal plasma lipid status. Common lipid abnormalities include elevated levels of total cholesterol, LDL-cholesterol, lipoprotein (a), triglyceride, HDL-cholesterol and a preponderance of small dense LDL particles. These abnormalities can be found alone or in combination. Most patients with atherosclerotic vascular disease have some form of dyslipidemia, even though their total cholesterol may not differ significantly from normal values. 35-40% of all CVD cases occur in patients with normal total cholesterol levels (< 5mmol/L, < 190mg/dl).

Total plasma cholesterol level should be below 5 mmol/L (190mg/dl) and LDL-cholesterol should below 3 mmol/L (115 mg/dl). For patients with clinically established CVD, patients with diabetes and asymptomatic people at high risk of developing CVD, treatment goals should be total cholesterol < 4.5 mmol/L (175mg/dl) and LDL-cholesterol < 2.5mmol/L (100mg/dl).

Treatment for HDL-cholesterol and triglycerides disorders are indicated if HDL-cholesterol values are < 1.0 mmol/L (<40mg/dl) in men and < 1.2mmol/L (46mg/dl) in women and fasting triglycerides> 1.7mmol/L (150mg/dl).

Target cholesterol values according to European Guidelines for CVD prevention in clinical practice:

1. Target cholesterol levels for the general population:
   Total cholesterol< 5 mmol/L (190mg/dl)
   LDL-cholesterol < 3 mmol/L (115mg/dl)
   HDL-cholesterol >1.2mmol/L (46mg/dl) in women and > 1.0mmol/L (40mg/dl) in men
   Triglycerides 1.7mmol/L (150mg/dl) or < 1.7mmol/L (150mg/dl)
2. Target cholesterol levels for patients at high risk:
   Total cholesterol < 4.5 mmol/L (175mg/dl)
   LDL-cholesterol < 2.5 mmol/L (100mg/dl)
   HDL-cholesterol- in women >1.2mmol/L (46mg/dl) and in men>1.0 mmol/L (40mg/dl)
   Triglycerides <1.7mmol/L (150mg/dl)

Studies demonstrate an association between increased concentrations of cholesterol, especially LDL-cholesterol and advanced atherosclerosis. Association of HDL-cholesterol levels with atherosclerosis is often underestimated, partly because most studies address the need for statin therapy.

However noted that the increased concentration of lipoprotein (a), Lp (a), a special kind of particles that have no metabolic closer ties with other lipoproteins, a risk factor for coronary heart disease as well as increased LDL-cholesterol. To explains the structural similarity glycoprotein (a) which is a major apoprotein of these particles with plasminogen and content of cholesterol and apoprotein B in these particles. These particles can inhibit fibrinolysis and promote competitive thrombogenesis by inhibiting binding of plasminogen for its binding sites on endothelium. The importance of risk factors is similar to smoking.

Dyslipidemia is a disorder of lipoprotein metabolism, caused by their excessive or otherwise, insufficient production. Disturbances characteristic of dyslipidemia include elevated levels of triglycerides (hypertriglyceridemia), decreased levels of HDL-cholesterol, elevated levels of LDL-cholesterol, lower LDL/HDL ratio and elevated levels of free fatty acids. Dyslipidemia is a heterogeneous disorder of complex etiology. The causes of dyslipidemia may be a primary and secondary. Primary causes include hereditary factors such as the deficit for the LDL receptor or apoprotein B involved in binding LDL particles to LDL receptor. In practice, the primary causes account for only a small part of cases, with predominance of secondary causes such as obesity, high fat intake, physical inactivity, smoking, diabetes and hypothyroidism.

Dyslipidemia, especially elevated concentration of LDL-cholesterol and decreased HDL-cholesterol, along with high blood pressure significantly contribute to wear-accelerated development of atherosclerosis, a condition in which fat, calcium and cellular degradation products accumulate along the walls of arteries forming atherosclerotic plaque. Over time, the plaque increases by reducing the diameter of blood vessels, its elasticity and therefore blood flow. Result of decreased elasticity can be ruptured blood vessels leading to cardiovascular diseases such as coronary heart disease or cerebrovascular disease.

A fasting lipoprotein profile, consisting of total cholesterol, LDL-cholesterol and triglycerides should be obtained in all adults over 20 and repeated at least once every 5 years. Blood samples should be drawn after 9-12 hour fast while the person is in a steady-absence of active weight loss, acute illness, recent trauma or surgery, pregnancy or recent change in diet. To ensure reliable measurements, blood samples should send to a laboratory recognized by an established standard program.

Once a dyslipidemia is diagnosed, a history, physical examination, and basic laboratory tests should be performed to screen for secondary cause of dyslipidemia, including diet, medications, alcohol abuse, diabetes, hypothyroidism, nephritic syndrome, chronic renal failure and obstructive liver disease. Raised cholesterol and free fatty acid levels in the blood represent a further risk factor for development of atherosclerosis and CHD. The strong relationship between LDL-cholesterol and CVD mandates intensive lowering of LDL-cholesterol thus reducing cardiovascular morbidity and mortality. Elevated levels of total cholesterol and LDL-cholesterol and low levels of HDL-cholesterol are major modifiable lipid risk factors for CVD and other forms of atherosclerotic vascular disease. It is estimated that for each 1% decrease in LDL-cholesterol and for each 1% increases HDL-cholesterol, the risk for cardiovascular events is reduced by 2% and 3%, respectively. Other important modifiable risk factors for CVD include elevated levels of triglyceride, lipoprotein(a), small dense LDL particles, homocysteine, C-reactive protein (CRP), fibrinogen and lipoprotein-associated phospholipase A2 (Lp-PLA2).

The frequent occurrence of raised blood lipid values in the western industrials and countries is attributable to a diet, which is high in fats, calories and carbohydrates and low in dietary fiber in combination with relatively little exercise. Blood lipids are bound to transport proteins in blood. Of particular interest in this respect is what known as the VLDL (very low-density lipoprotein) lipoprotein transport molecule, the LDL (low-density lipoprotein) lipoprotein transport molecule and the HDL (high-density lipoprotein) lipoprotein transport molecule. These terms describe the physical-chemical properties of the molecules and serve to distinguish between them when analyzing lipids in laboratory.

The LDL molecules carry more than 60-70% of the cholesterol bound in the blood and are therefore the „risk molecule" for atherosclerosis. The HDL molecule carries about 35% of the cholesterol and above all captures the cholesterol, which passes from the tissues into the blood. Ultimately, the VLDL molecules carry only 10-15% of total cholesterol and most of the free fatty acids.

The risk of the premature development of general atherosclerotic condition increases with the proportion of LDL and VLDL molecules in the blood and decreases with the level of the HDL content. In general, a reduction in total cholesterol, or LDL fraction, leads to a reduction of 2 to 3% of the risk of developing CHD. Assessment of the risk of each individual patient requires individual assessment of each component of blood lipids, and the determination of total cholesterol and of the free fatty acids. The HDL values are about 10-20% higher in women than men of all ages. They increase with regular participation in sports, but are lower in smokers, overweight and diabetics. The other known risk factors are also reflected by the individual blood lipid values.

2.2.2 Identification of genetic dyslipidemia

If severe hypercholesterolemia is present (total cholesterol > 7.7mmol/L or > 300mg/dl) or a genetic disorder is discovered, a family history and measurement of cholesterol in other family members is indicated.

2.2.3 Hyperlipidemia

Hyperlipidemia is a type of lipid disorder consisting of hypercholesterolemia and hypertriglyceridemia and is marked by increased lipids concentration in the blood. It is classified in six classes (according to Frederickson). For clinical purpose, it is divided into primary, or familial hyperlipidemia caused by genetic factors and secondary (acquired) hyperlipidemia, which arise because of liver disease, diabetes or thyroid gland disorder. Other important risk factors for the occurrence of secondary hyperlipidemia are the use of some medications and birth control pills. Although part of hyperlipidemia is due to genetic reasons, the majority of secondary hyperlipidemias occurs as the effects of lifestyle, inadequate physical activity and improper and diet. One should borne in mind that, despite all the pathology caused by hyperlipidaemia, fats are essential for normal functioning of the organism.

2.2.3.1 Hypercholesterolemia

Hypercholesterolemia or increased blood cholesterol level found in diseases such as hepatitis, renal disease, hypothyroidism and diabetes. Hypercholesterolemia is often a consequence of inadequate nutrition, rich in saturated fatty acids. Therefore, dietary changes, increased physical activity and finally pharmacological therapy are advised for people with elevated cholesterol levels in blood. Unfortunately, most of the blood cholesterol is produced in liver so lifestyle changes can lower cholesterol level no more than 15%. Therefore, therapy in indicated in cases of insufficient results from diet. Studies show that high levels of total cholesterol and LDL-cholesterol are one of the major causes of cardiovascular diseases and maintaining proper LDL/HDL ratio reduces the risk of CVD.

2.2.3.2 Hypertrygliceridemia

Hypertriglyceridemia is elevated level of triglycerides, with normal LDL-cholesterol level. Hypertriglyceridemia usually occurs as results of poor eating habits and inadequate physical activity and is common in obese people. Basic recommendation in the triglyceride lowering diets are reducing fat intake up to 15% of total calories (fatty meat, fried foods, replacing animal fat with vegetable), reducing the amount of carbohydrates up to 55% of total daily caloric intake, selection of complex carbohydrates (cereals, pasta, potatoes) and intake of foods rich in omega-3 fatty acids (fish, fish oil).

2.2.3.3 Combined hyperlipidemia

There are often combined hyperlipidemias with the elevated blood levels of both cholesterol and triglycerides. It can be result of bad habits and obesity, genetic predisposition or as a result of certain diseases and condition. It also represents major risk for coronary heart disease.

2.2.4 Lipoproteins and lipoproteins components

Lp (a)-Lp little is low-density lipoprotein that binds an additional protein called lipoprotein a. High concentration Lp (a) increases the risk of atherosclerosis.

Apolipoprotein A is the main components of HDL-cholesterol. Lower values of Apo A and low HDL-cholesterol is associated with increased risk of atherosclerosis.

Apoliprotein B is a major component of LDL, IDL, and VLDL apoB chylomicrons. Therefore, it is located in atherogenic lipoproteins. The concentration of apoB is a direct of concentration of atherogenic lipoproteins in plasma. This parameter is a useful indicator of atherosclerosis in patients with hypertriglyceridemia and with normal LDL-cholesterol.

2.2.5 Severe familial hyperlipidemias

Familial hypercholesterolemia (FH) is characterized by hypercholesterolemia and associated with elevated levels LDL-cholesterol, xanthomata, premature coronary heart disease with positive family history. CVD occur in men between 30-50 years, in women 50-70 years. It is present in 5-10 % of individuals with CVD at age below 55 years.

Familial Combined hyperlipidemia (FCH) is this most common among severe hyperlipidemia, with the prevalence of 1/100 (the most common clinically relevant genetic disorder).

2.3 Diabetes mellitus, insulin resistance and metabolic syndrome

2.3.1 Diabetes mellitus

Diabetes mellitus, both type 1 and type 2, is also a major risk factor for cardiovascular disease. Hyperlipoproteinemia, hypertriglyceridemia in particular, i.e. elevated levels of very-low density lipoprotein (VLDL) particles and atherogenic LDL deriving from VLDL, with concurrent decrease in the level of protective HDL particles are quite common in diabetic patients. LDL particles that undergo no enzymatic glucosylation due to elevated blood glucose undergo prompt phagocytosis by macrophages, thus stimulating atherogenesis. In addition, hyperinsulinemia causes damage to vascular endothelium.

Since diabetes is one of the major modifiable risk factor for CVD, its' prevention in one of the main goals of modern cardiovascular medicine. Inadequate physical activity decreases the concentration of HDL, whereas obesity is associated with hyperglycaemia and hyperinsulinemia. CHD is the major threat to modern society and, according to estimations; it will remain so at least by 2020. Therefore, all efforts invested in the study of cardiovascular disease are fully justified. In line with this, recording and analysis of the prevalence of risk factors for cardiovascular disease as the most common cause of CVD.

Progression to diabetes can be prevented or delayed by lifestyle intervention in individuals with impaired glucose tolerance. In patient with type 1 and type 2 diabetes, good metabolic control prevents microvascular complications and can prevent cardiovascular events. In type 1 diabetes, glucose control requires appropriate insulin therapy and concomitant professional dietary therapy. In type 2 diabetes, professional dietary advice, reduction of overweight and increased physical activity should be the first treatment aiming at good glucose control. Treatment goals for blood pressure and lipids are generally more ambitions in patient with diabetes (see previous sections).

Diabetes is also a very important CVD risk factor. It is known that the frequency and intensity of artery atherosclerosis is higher in diabetes, especially type 2. Three quarters of diabetic patients die from diseases caused by atherosclerosis, especially coronary artery disease and ischemic stroke. Only long-term reduction of glucose level decreases a risk of atherosclerosis. The men with proven glucose intolerance have even 50% higher risk of coronary heart disease than men with normal test submission glucose. Risk is even twice higher in women. Mortality from CVD in diabetic's disease is ten times higher than in people who have no diabetes. In diabetic's hyperlipoprotenemia, particularly hypertriglyceridemia, is more common, the amount VDLD-particles is higher, more atherogenic LDL-particles are generated by VLDL-particles degradation and the amount of protective HDL-particles is reduced. Macrophages phagocytes LDL- particles faster, due to increased amounts of glucose in the blood promoting non-enzymatic glycosylation, thus stimulating atherogenesis. Altered metabolisms of glycosaminoglycans in diabetic patients are also important for the increased incidence of hyperglycaemia-related atherosclerotic changes. Hyperglycemia, similar to LDL-cholesterol and VLDL-cholesterol in plasma, slows down the regeneration of endothelial cells, encouraging atherogenesis. Hyperglycemia acts as oxidant, accelerating oxidation of LDL-cholesterol particles, partially by reducing concentrations of vitamin C. No enzymatic glucosylation of collagen, accelerated by hyperglycaemia also stimulates platelet aggregation and thus atherogenesis. Altered collagen strongly binds LDL-particles. Diabetic platelets synthesize more thromboxane and endothelial cells syntheses less prostacyclin, also contributing to thrombocyte aggregation. Elevated concentrations of insulin promote atherogenesis, because insulin stimulates migration of smooth muscle cells from media into the intimae, their proliferation at the site of endothelial injury and activity of their receptors for LDL-cholesterol. It is widely known that many diabetics, particularly those with type 2 are overweight, with hyperinsulinemia due to peripheral vascular tissue resistance to insulin. Many of them have hypertension, which also contributes to the rapid atherosclerosis. Glucose intolerance or insulin resistance and consequent hyperinsulinemia is associated with central obesity type, hypertension, elevated triglycerides and decreased HDL-cholesterol, making up metabolic syndrome, which further increases the risk of atherosclerosis. Since diabetics have a much greater, risk than others patients, diabetic patient with another risk factor, particularly hyperlipidemia, demands more aggressive approach.

Diabetes mellitus is metabolic disorder characterized by chronic hyperglycaemia with disturbances of carbohydrate, fat and protein metabolism resulting from defects of insulin secretion, insulin action or a combination of both. The etiological classification has proposed by the WHO in 1999. There are 4 specific categories:

1. Type I diabetes characterized by an absolute insulin deficiency of autoimmune or idiopathic nature. Typically, in the vast majority of cases it occurs at younger age.
2. Type 2 diabetes characterized by a relative insulin deficiency coupled with an insulin resistance state. It includes over 90% the diabetic states developing after middle age. This diabetic state is often seen in people with visceral obesity and metabolic syndrome.
3. Gestational diabetes developing during pregnancy and in most cases disappearing after delivery. 60-70% of these patients will progress to diabetes during their life.
4. Other particular forms of diabetes include the clinical conditions secondary to diseases of exocrine pancreas (inflammation, trauma, neoplasm, and pancreatectomy) and endocrine system (Syndrome Cushing, phaeochromocytoma, acromegalia). It also includes genetic defects of beta cells and drug-induced diabetic states, such as those trigged by cortisone, antidepressants, beta-blockers and thiazide diuretics.

The clinical classification is based on criteria proposed by the WHO in 1999. In addition, The American Society of Diabetology (ADA, 2003.). The WHO recommendations for glucometabolic classification based on measuring both fasting and two hour post-load glucose concentrations and recommend that a standardized 75g glucose tolerance test (OGTT) should be performed in the absence of overt hyperglycaemia. Glycated haemoglobin (HBA1c) is useful measure of metabolic control and the efficacy of glucose lowering treatment in people with diabetes. It presents a mean value of blood glucose during the preceding six to eight weeks (life span of erythrocytes). HBA1c not recommended as a diagnostic test for diabetes. Because normal values do not exclude diabetes or impaired glucose tolerance. The approach for early detection of diabetes and people in risk of acquiring diabetes is measuring of blood glucose in people who are at risk due to their demographic and clinical characteristics. Collecting questionnaire-based information on etiological factors for type 2 diabetes is necessary. Glycaemia testing (OGTT) is always necessary as a secondary step to accurately defined impaired glucose homeostasis. Glucometabolic abnormalities are common in patients with CVD and an OGTT should carry out in them. In the general population the appropriate strategy is to start with risk assessment as the primary screening tool combined with subsequent glucose testing (OGTT) of individuals identified to be at high risk. The relationship between hyperglycaemia and CVD should be seen as continuum. For each 1% increase of HBA1c there is defined increased risk for CVD. The risk of CVD for people with overt diabetes increased by two to three times for men and three to five times for women compared with people without diabetes. In type 1 diabetic patients prevalence of CVD amounts to 10% with a pronounced increase when diabetic nephropathy is detected. In type 2 diabetic patients prevalence of CVD is higher and almost similar to that displayed by patients with history of a previous myocardial infarction. Cardiovascular complications have a higher adverse impact on mortality in type 2 than type 1 diabetes (55% vs. 44%). It is still debated whether asymptomatic hyperglycaemia is associated with an increased risk of coronary events. Information on post-prandial (post-load) glucose also predicts increased cardiovascular risk in subjects with normal fasting glucose levels. The most common cause of death in adults with diabetes is CVD. Their risk is two to three times higher than that among people without diabetes. The combination of type 2 diabetes and previous CAD identifies patients with particularly high risk for coronary deaths. The relative effect of diabetes is lager in women than men (Table 3).

Elevated 2-hour post-load plasma glucose has much bigger impact on cardiovascular risk than fasting glucose. For major cardiovascular risk factors, mortality and cardiovascular morbidity are predicted by hyperglycaemia itself. Elevated blood glucose levels have an adverse impact on cardiovascular risk profile by decreasing vascular function (in particular endothelial function) and reducing nitric oxide bioavailability.

2.3.2 Insulin resistance

Insulin resistance contributes to the development and progression of several of the above-mentioned abnormalities. This is because the insulin-resistance state (and the related hyperinsulinemic condition) impairs the endothelium-dependent vasodilatation and promotes, through the activation of specific protein-kinase subfamilies, the development and progression of the vascular inflammatory and atherogenic process.

2.3.3 The metabolic syndrome

Dyslipidemia of diabetic patient is characterized by moderate hypertriglyceridemia, low HDL-cholesterol and impaired post-prandial lipid response. The prevalence of dyslipidemia

Glucometabolic category	Source	Classification criteria
Normal glucose regulation (NGR)	WHO	FPG < 6.1 (110) + 2 h PG < 7.8 (140)
	ADA (1997)	FPG < 6.1 (110)
	ADA (2003)	FPG < 5.6 (100)
Impaired fasting glucose (IFG)	WHO	FPG ≥ 6.1 (110) and < 7.0 (126) + 2 h PG < 7.8 (140)
	ADA (1997)	FPG ≥ 6.1 (110) and < 7.0 (126)
	ADA (2003)	FPG ≥ 5.6 (100) and < 7.0 (126)
Impaired glucose tolerance (IGT)	WHO	FPG < 7.0 (126) + 2 h PG ≥ 7.8 and < 11.1 (200)
Impaired glucose homeostasis (IGH)	WHO	IFG or IGT
Diabetes mellitus	WHO	FPG ≥ 7.0 (126) or 2 h PG ≥ 11.1 (200)
	ADA (1997)	FPG ≥ 7.0 (126)
	ADA (2003)	FPG ≥ 7.0 (126)

Table 3. Criteria used for glucometabolic classification from WHO (1999 and 2006) and ADA (1997 and 2003). Abbreviations: FPG – fasting plasma glucose, PG – postprandial glucose. Units are mmol/l and mg/dl (in brackets)

is two/three times greater in patients with glucose intolerance and diabetes, compared to metabolically healthy subjects. LDL-cholesterol values participate in determining the cardiovascular risk. The evidence that a raise in LDL-cholesterol amounting to 1.0mmol/L (38.7mg/dl) is associated with a 57% elevation in cardiovascular events rate confirms this. Similar data have reported for low HDL-cholesterol. It is still uncertain whether the relationship between plasma triglycerides and vascular risk is independent from other metabolic factors (so called hyperinsulinemic cluster).

There has been an interest in clustering factors, each one associated with increased risk for CVD, together in the metabolic syndrome. It was debated whether such clustering represents a disease entity in its own, but it helps identifying individuals at high risk for cardiovascular disease and type 2 diabetes. Currently there are several definitions. The International Federation of Diabetes has issued the most recent. The pathogenesis of the metabolic syndrome and its components is complex and not yet well understood. However, central obesity and insulin resistance are important causative factors. Abdominal circumference and waist to hip ratio (W/H) is very useful screening factors for the metabolic syndrome, much more associated with metabolic risk then commonly used body mass index.

International Diabetes Federation-Metabolic Syndrome Definition

- Central Obesity (defined as waist circumference > 94 cm for European men and >80 cm for European women, with ethnicity specific values for other groups).

In addition, any two of the following four factors:

- Raised TG level :> 1.7 mmol/L (150 mg/dl), or specific treatment for this lipid abnormality.
- Reduced HDL cholesterol :< 1.0 mmol/L (40 mg/dl) in males and < 1.2 mmol/L (50 mg/dl) in females, or specific treatment for this lipid abnormality.
- Raised blood pressure: systolic BP >130 or diastolic BP >85 mmHg, or treatment of previously diagnosed hypertension.
- Raised fasting plasma glucose (FPG)> 5.6 mmol/L (100mg/dl) or previously diagnosed type 2 diabetes.

If glucose level is above 5.6 mmol/L or 100mg/dl, OGTT is strongly recommended but is not necessary to define presence of the syndrome.

Compared to the opinions expressed by other Guidelines and Scientific Societies, the European Guidelines seem to take a conservative position on the clinical impact of cardiovascular risk profile in patients with metabolic syndrome. This is partially because the two Societies are still waiting for further evidence.

The diabetogenic risk of patients with CVD is super imposable to the one characterizing subjects with obesity or metabolic syndrome. Patient with a high cardiovascular risk a glucose intolerance state may be responsible for the elevated prevalence of sudden death. Adequate control of postprandial hyperglycaemia has a favourable impact on cardiovascular and all-cause mortality. The elevated cardiovascular risk profile displayed by the diabetic patient depends not only on the glycaemia (and insulin) abnormality but also, and largely, on the development and progression of the atherogenic vascular process. The mechanisms include oxidative stress, the dyslipdemic state and the pro-atherogenic process.

1. Oxidative stress represents one of the cornerstones of the endothelial dysfunction as well as of the atherogenic process, but clinical studies are still inconclusive on this issue and do not to clarify whether and to what extent anti-oxidative drugs have a favourable therapeutic impact on the atherosclerotic process.
2. Dyslipidaemic state - lipid disorders classically described in diabetes include a elevated triglycerides and LDL and decreased HDL levels. Recent evidences support the role of free fatty acids (whose plasma concentrations increased in diabetes) in favouring the atherogenic process. Along with free fatty acids, another proatherogenic factor is the accumulation of triglyceride-rich lipoproteins, due to a reduced clearance by lipoprotein lipases.
3. Pro-atherogenic process and thrombosis - hyperglycaemia and insulin resistance exert adverse effects on thrombosis and coagulation by altering platelet function. Key features of the altered thrombosis process are the increased expression of glycoproteins, overproduction of fibrinogen, thrombin and von Willebrand factor as well as the reduction in endogenous anticoagulants (thrombomodulin and protein C).
4. The pathophysiological alterations responsible for the increased atherogenic risk, typical of the diabetic state are multifaceted. Several of these alterations are shared by the metabolic syndrome, which also includes glycaemia abnormalities as a key patho-physiological feature.

Diabetes doubles the probability of developing CHD or a cardiovascular disease in general. Death from the consequences of CHD increases by a factor of four to six. Next to occlusive diseases of the vessels of the lower extremities, (peripheral arterial occlusive vascular disease) coronary heart disease is the most frequent complication in diabetes. The presence of additional risk factors, such as obesity, lipometabolic disorders, high blood pressure or smoking, endangers diabetics more than any other patient group.

Unfortunately, a great deal is still unclear regarding the effects of diabetes on the development and course of CHD.

2.4 Obesity and overweight

Many people believe that central or abdominal type of obesity is not an independent risk factor, but is associated with hypertension, diabetes and dyslipidemia. In extremely obese persons, low level of protective HDL-cholesterol is an independent risk factor for the hyperinsulinemia combined with hyperglycaemia. Insufficient physical activity is another major risk factors. Regular physical activity significantly reduces the incidence of coronary artery disease and myocardial infarction. Current recommends daily exercise, swimming, walking, cycling and other physical activity Regular physical activity slightly lower blood pressure, affects weight loss, improves glucose tolerance and exerts a positive effect on the blood clotting system. Physical activity stimulates rise in HDL-cholesterol concentration, and reduces triglycerides level in the blood. The most common reason for the accumulation of excessive weight is a sedentary lifestyle and unhealthy diet. Obesity is often perceived as a necessary companion of the thirties and forties. Proper nutrition, education and moderate physical activity can solve most of these problems so that education and prevention offers a solution for obesity and overweight. Adipose tissue on the hips and abdomen is deleterious only to our appearance and confidence, because it causes hormonal imbalance. Adipose tissue in obese people is the biggest endocrine organ in the body. Secretion of various hormones (the most important leptin), leads to insulin resistance and the occurrence of type 2 diabetes. Weight gain increases proportionately with blood pressure and all its harmful effects on the walls of blood vessels. Excessive calories intakes, which are, not spend but stored in our body as fat. It is believed that cholesterol and fatty acids in the blood have a crucial effect on the development of atherosclerotic plaques in blood vessels. Obesity burdens the entire organism, making obese people jumpy and easily fatigued. Large deposits of fat in the abdomen decrease lung capacity because the chest cannot expand of the lungs normally. This causes shortness of breath, especially at night due to a horizontal body position. Often awakening because of shortness of breath disturbs the normal structure of sleep and causes sleep deprivation and chronic fatigue. Consequently, obese people are less efficient at work and have much more incidence of bad mood and depression.

Today, definition of overweight and obesity is made according to by Body Mass Index (BMI), representing the ratio of body weight and body height squared. Values of BMI range from 18.5 to more of 30. BMI less than 18.5 indicates malnutrition, optimal values ranging from 18.5 to 24.9, overweight point value of 25 to 30 and a value greater than 30 indicate obesity and represent a serious health risk. Being overweight has a negative effect on other risk factors such as high blood pressure, immobility, lipometabolic disorders and a tendency to diabetes. However, being overweight by approximately 10% above the ideal weight, when taken into consideration as an independent risk factor, has great significance for the development of cardiovascular diseases, particularly in people below the age of 50. People who throughout their lives remain approximately 20% overweight have about a 50% greater risk of developing CVD than those who are of normal waist 88 cm in women. Avoiding overweight or reducing existing overweight is important. Weight reduction is strongly recommended for obese people (BMI> 30 kg/m2) or overweight individuals (BMI > 25 and > 30 kg/m2) and for those with increased abdominal fat as indicated by waist circumference >102 cm in men and > 88 cm in women. Restriction of total caloric intake and regular practice of physical exercise should advise in overweight and obese patients.

2.5 Mental stress

Nowadays it is believed that lack of social support and social isolation, unemployment, stress at work with an indefinite time, night work, family conflicts and depression also present an important risk factors. Such people are more likely to smoke, consume large quantities of alcohol and unhealthy food. The people with lower socio-economic status, lower education, who hold lower-paying jobs are three times more likely to suffer from coronary disease. Permanent alertness of the autonomic nervous system and hypothalamus-pituitary-adrenal axis, leads to increased blood pressure, changes in endothelial function and blood coagulation system and proinflammatory stimulus, which encourages atherogenesis.

Mental stress and depression both predispose to increased vascular risk and from a clinician's perspective should be considered as modifiable risk factors. The adrenergic stimulation during mental stress can augment myocardial oxygen requirements and aggravate myocardial ischemia. Mental stress can cause coronary vasoconstriction, particularly in atherosclerotic coronary arteries and hence can influence myocardial oxygen supply as well. Recent studies have further linked mental stress to platelet and endothelial dysfunction, the metabolic syndrome and the induction of ventricular arrhythmias.

Acute stress such (studied in cases of great natural disasters) has long been recognized as a risk factor for coronary events. More recently, work-related stress has gained recognition as a source of vascular risk. Work stress has two components: job strain (which combines high work demands and low job control) and effort-reward imbalance (which more closely reflects economic factors in the workplace). Both components are associated with an approximate doubling of risk for myocardial infarction and stroke in European and Japanese populations. Other psychological metrics, including anger and hostility scales, have also been associated with elevated vascular risk.

Clinical depression strongly predicts coronary heart disease. In meta-analysis of studies involving initially healthy individuals, those with depression had a significantly higher risk of developing coronary disease during follow-up, with clinical depression being more important than depressive mood. While depression is also associated with an increased prevalence of hypertension, smoking and lack of physical activity, the effects of depression on overall risk remain after adjusting for these and other traditional risk factors. Thus, findings that depressed individuals also have increased platelet activation, elevated levels of high sensitive C-reactive protein (hsCRP), and decreased heart rate variability support depression as an independent predictor of cardiovascular events. Onset of depression after myocardial infarction is common and predicts cardiovascular mortality independent of cardiac disease severity. Whether therapy for post infarction depression reduces recurrent event rates remains controversial and open to research.

2.5.1 Stress and the heart

When organism is under stress, secretion of stress hormones adrenaline and noradrenalin strains the heart. This can gradually lead to cardiac arrhythmias, angina pectoris on exertion and eventually myocardial infarction. Additional risk factors for such persons are unhealthy diet, excessive smoking and alcohol consumption.

2.6 Lack of physical activity

Regular physical activity protects against the onset of cardiovascular disorders. Inactive people have about twice the risk of developing a vascular disease than people who are active. Regular physical activity, whether pursuing a sport or just in the form of working in the garden, improves the heart muscle oxygenation its function, delays ageing of the vessels and protects against cardiac arrhythmias. The duration, intensity and frequency of the activity must be sufficient to achieve a training effect.

Physical exercise also has a beneficial effect on other risk factors: reduced weight, improved glucose tolerance in diabetes and normalized blood lipid and lowering of blood pressure.

People with risk factors for CHD who have previously not undertaken any sports should only do so after advice from a physician because unaccustomed exertion in the presence of underlying CHD can lead to sudden cardiac death.

2.7 Personality structure and social environment

The attempt of psychologists to establish a personality structure, which is particularly at risk of developing coronary heart disease, has led to definition of the „type A"behavior pattern. „Type A "personalities are characterized by latent aggression, impatience, competitive thoughts, time pressure in everyday life and brusqueness in the way they speak and behave. Chronically suppressed hostile behaviour towards others and feelings of fury appear to be linked to particular disadvantage. One reason for this could be that an unbalanced mental state leads to a permanent state of stress. This reflected in particularly by increased production of catecholamine, the stress hormones of the body.

2.8 Smoking cigarettes and nicotine

Nicotine is a powerful poison that causes dependency. In the cardiovascular system, heart rate and blood pressure raise with narrowing of blood vessels. Nicotine exerts additional adverse effect on the nervous system, heart, blood vessels, kidney, gastrointestinal tract and genital organs.

2.8.1 Cigarette smoking

Cigarette smoking increases LDL and decreases HDL, also increasing carbon monoxide in serum, thus leading to endothelial hypoxia and potentially to vasoconstriction of the already narrowed atherosclerotic arteries. Cigarette smoking can also enhance platelet activity, which in turn may lead to the formation of thrombus and an increase in plasma fibrin and hematocrit, thus contributing to blood viscosity.

Beyond acute unfavourable effects on blood pressure, sympathetic tone and a reduction in myocardial oxygen supply, smoking affects atherotrombosis by several other mechanisms. In addition to accelerating atherosclerotic progression, long-term smoking may enhance oxidation of LDL-cholesterol and impairs endothelium-dependent coronary artery vasodilatation. This latter effect has been directly linked to dysfunctional endothelial nitric oxide biosynthesis following chronic as well as acute cigarette consumption. In addition, smoking has adverse haemostatic and inflammatory effects, including increased levels of hsCRP (high-sensitivity C-reactive protein) soluble intercellular adhesion molecule-1 (ICAM-1), fibrinogen and homocysteine. Smoking is associated with spontaneous platelet aggregation, increased monocyte adhesion to endothelial cells and adverse alterations in endothelial derived fibrinolytic and antithrombotic factors, including tissue-type plasminogen activator and tissue pathway factor inhibitor. Compared with non-smokers, smokers have increased prevalence of coronary spasm and may have reduced thresholds for ventricular arrhythmia. Accumulating evidence suggest that insulin resistance represents an additional mechanistic link between smoking and premature atherosclerosis. Smoking is a strong risk factor for the development of arteriosclerosis and CHD. There is a dose-related connection between the number of cigarettes smoked, the number of years of smoking and the risk of the development of cardiovascular disease. Habitual smokers have twice the risk of developing a cardiovascular disorder and three times the risk of sudden cardiac death. Cigar and pipe smokers also exposed to an increased risk. Various factors contribute to the negative effects of smoking on health: the damaging effect on the endothelium, the negative change in blood lipid values, increased propensity to thrombosis (particularly in women also on oral hormonal contraception), increased propensity to heart rhythm disturbances and the associated pulmonary diseases, which involve the heart consequently. Usage of oral hormonal contraception containing estrogen compounds is not recommended in smokers. If there is already underlying CHD, smoking has particularly negative consequences, because the red blood pigment (haemoglobin) of smokers cannot supply sufficient oxygen to the heart muscle cells when the coronary vessels are constricted. Symptoms of angina pectoris are particularly likely to occur during exertion in smokers with CHD. With regard to prevention, it is important that the risk of becoming ill from a cardiovascular disorder is reduced to that of a non-smoker after just one year of abstaining from nicotine. Unfortunately, this does not apply to the same extent for risk of a former smoker from developing cancer or a chronic pulmonary disease.

2.8.2 Second hand smoke exposure

Second hand smoke exposure is the risk factor when person experiences more than 1 hour of passive smoke exposure per week.

2.9 C-reactive protein (CRP)

Inflammation characterizes all phases of atherotrombosis and provides a critical physiological link between plaque formation and acute rupture, leading to occlusion and infarction.

CRP is a circulating member of the pentraxin family and plays a major role in the human innate immune response. It is primarily produced in the liver; recent data indicate that cells within human coronary arteries, particularly in the atherosclerotic intimae, can synthesise CRP. More than being a marker of inflammation, CRP may influence directly vascular vulnerability through several mechanisms, including enhanced expression of local adhesion molecules, increased expression of endothelial PAI-1 (plasminogen activator inhibitor), reduced endothelial nitric oxide bioactivity, altered LDL uptake by macrophages and co localization with complement within atherosclerotic lesions. The expression of human CRP in CRP transgenic mice directly enhances intravascular thrombosis and accelerates atherogenesis. In primary prevention, CRP, when measured with hsCRP, strongly and independently predicts risk of myocardial infarction, stroke, peripheral arterial disease and sudden cardiac death even among apparently healthy individuals. These data apply to women as well as to men across all age levels and consistently to diverse populations. Hs-CRP is an independent marker of risk and, in those judged at intermediate risk by global risk assessment, measurement of hs-CRP may help direct further evaluation and therapy in the primary prevention of cardiovascular disease. The benefits of such therapy based on this strategy remain uncertain. In patients with stable coronary disease or acute coronary syndromes, hs-CRP measurement may be useful as an independent marker of prognosis for recurrent events, including death, myocardial infarction, and restenosis after percutaneous coronary intervention (PCI). The benefits of therapy based on this strategy remain uncertain. Hs-CRP levels, using standardized assays, should categorize patients into one of three relative risk categories: low risk < 1.0mg/L; average risk 1.0-3.0 mg/L; high risk > 3.0mg/L. Measurement of hs-CRP should be done twice (averaging results), optimally two weeks apart, fasting or no fasting in metabolically stable patients. If hs-CRP level is > 10mg/L, the test should repeat and the patient examined for sources of infection or inflammation. The entire adult population should not screen for hs-CRP for cardiovascular risk assessment, not should hs-CRP levels used to determine preventive measures for secondary prevention or for patients with acute coronary syndromes. CRP was relatively moderate predictor of CVD risk an added only marginally to the prediction of CVD risk based on established risk factors.

2.10 Fibrinogen

Increased plasma fibrinogen is a risk factor because it increases blood viscosity and platelet aggregation and promotes thrombogenesis. More over fibrinogen is the acute phase reactant, and serves as a marker of inflammation, an important component of atherogenesis. Plasma fibrinogen influences platelet aggregations and blood viscosity, interacts with plasminogen binding and in combination with thrombin, mediates the final step in clot formation and the response to vascular injury. In addition, fibrinogen associates positively with age, obesity, smoking cigarettes, diabetes and LDL-cholesterol level and inversely with HDL-cholesterol level, alcohol use physical activity and exercise level. Fibrinogen level, like CRP, an acute phase reactant, increases during inflammatory responses. Studies found no significant positive associations between fibrinogen levels and future risk of cardiovascular events.

2.11 Imunoreactivity

Imunoreactivity could also be an important factor in the development of endothelial damage and thus atherosclerosis development. It is supported by the finding of the accumulated lipids in the affected arterioles of patients with dermatomyositis, systemic lupus erythematosus, scleroderma and rheumatoid arthritis. Atherosclerosis is more common after the transplantation of organs; it also explains the deposition of immune complexes in the walls of arteries and their damage.

2.12 Homocysteine

Increased homocysteine level is also a risk factor for atherosclerosis. People with levels of homocysteine higher than 12 mmol/L have twice the risk of myocardial infarction regardless of sex. Homocysteine acts proatherogenically because it changes the function of the endothelium and promotes the oxidation of LDL.

Homocysteine is a sulfhydryl-containing amino acid derived from the demethylastion of dietary methionine. Patient with rare inherited defects of methionine metabolism can develop severe hyperhomocysteinemia (plasma level >100µmol/L) and have markedly elevated risk of premature atherothrombosis as well as venous thromboembolism. The mechanisms that account for these effects remain uncertain but include endothelial dysfunction, accelerated oxidation of LDL-cholesterol, impairment of flow-mediated endothelial-derived relaxing factor with subsequent reduction in arterial vasodilatation,

platelet activation, increased expression of monocyte chemoattractant protein (MCP-1) and interleukin-8 leading to a proinflammatory response and oxidative stress.
Measurement of homocysteine levels should reserve for individuals with atherosclerosis at a young age or out of proportion to established risk factors. Clinical trials have not shown that intervention to lower homocysteine levels reduces CVD events.

2.13 Albuminuria

Albuminuria is a result of kidney glomerular damage; increased albuminuria indicates a higher risk of progression of kidney disease. Hypertension and albuminuria are independent factors affecting long-term reduction of kidney function. Renal disease is both a cause and consequence of hypertension. Treating arterial hypertension reduces cardiovascular risk and risk of kidney damage. Reducing albuminuria also reduces total cardiovascular risk and kidney damage.

2.14 Hyperuricemia

Hyperuricemia is a high value of serum uric acid in blood: higher of 360 μmol/L (6 mg/dl) for women and 400 μmol/L (6.8 mg/dl) for men. It has double effect: damages the endothelium and smooth muscle cells of blood vessels and acts as an oxidant. Epidemiologic study found an association between hyperuricemia and hypertension, renal disease and CVD.

3. Non-modifiable risk factors

3.1 Sex and age

3.1.1 Sex

It is well known that blood vessels age more rapidly in men than in women. As a result, women in their 50-es demonstrate significantly less advanced atherosclerotic changes then men of the same age. Only one of seven women aged between 45 and 64 have signs of coronary heart disease. After the age of 65, however, the frequency increases to one in three. Two thirds of women affected by CHD die because of the it. An increase in free fatty acids and blood cholesterol, high blood pressure, diabetes, nicotine and alcohol consumption promote the vessel ageing process in women as well. The epidemiological observation that before the menopause women are affected by CHD much less than men has led to the conclusion that the female sex hormone, estrogen, has a protective effect on the cardiovascular system. Data from clinical trials indicates a 35-50% reduction in the risk of developing CHD if estrogen supplemental treatment is undertaken.
This effect of estrogen is partially attributed to a hormone-induced increase in HDL-cholesterol blood lipid carrier protein and on the other to a reduction in the potentially vessel-damaging LDL-cholesterol blood lipid carrier protein, which is loaded predominantly with cholesterol. One should emphasize, however, that observed men and women should be exposed to the same risk factors. Before the start of the menopause women benefit from a relative protection from development of CHD due to the presence of the female sex hormone, estrogen. After the onset of the menopause, the relative risk for men and women equals. The administration of synthetic estrogens can, irrespective of the reasons why gynaecologists prescribe hormone treatment, also have the positive side effect of protecting against CVD.

Male sex is a risk factor that has been proven in numerous epidemiological studies, regardless of the higher incidence of other risk factors in men than in women. It known that the atherosclerotic changes, especially coronary arteries and blood vessels, come about 10 years later in women than in men. This is partly explained by the beneficial effects of estrogen on lipoproteins, because they increase HDL-cholesterol and reduce LDL-cholesterol and Lp(a), oxidation LDL-cholesterol, fibrinogen and homocysteine. Sex hormones may have direct effects on blood vessels because existence of receptors for androgens and estrogens on smooth muscle cells of the blood vessels has been proven. Even after menopause, cardiovascular risk is still significantly lower in women than in men of the same age. Nevertheless, in most developed countries cardiovascular diseases are the major causes of mortality in women, not only in men.

3.1.2 Menopause and hormonal therapy

Women who enter menopause early (before age 50) are three times more likely to have coronary disease. Although some earlier studies suggested that there is an association between taking oral hormonal contraception (OHC) and the occurrence of coronary disease, today we know that (OHC) usage presents cardiovascular risk only in women with additional risk factors, especially smoking cigarettes. Estrogen containing oral contraceptives stimulate liver production of VLDL-cholesterol and therefore LDL-cholesterol level in women who have previously known family hyperlipidemia. On the other hand, taking oral contraceptive with higher dose of estrogen causes an increase in HDL-cholesterol concentration and might be antiatherogenic, but it not scientifically proven. Although hormone replacement therapy in postmenopausal women have numerous benefits (control of vasomotor symptoms, prevention of osteoporosis, etc.), previous opinions about its positive effect on the prevention coronary disease, are no longer uniformly endorsed.

3.1.3 Age

The risk of developing coronary heart disease and suffering myocardial infarction increases with age for both sexes. However, atherosclerosis does not however begin abruptly. The signs of incipient coronary atherosclerosis can be apparent from a very early stage. Studies have shown that atherosclerotic transformation processes of aorta can become apparent even in three years old children. Thus, the coronary vessels are involved in this process from in patient's youth (20 or 30 years). Although age is an important factor, the probability of developing coronary heart disease varies according to the presence of the additional risk factors. The best estimate of the individual's risk is therefore provided by consideration of age in relation to other risk factors present. The observation that significant atherosclerotic changes in the coronary vessels can start very early in life emphasizes the need for prevention at an early stage.

3.2 Genetic factors

Genetic information can be divided into categories: data from family history, data on genotypes and phenotypes.

3.2.1 Family history (hereditary risk)

Heritage is considered a risk factor because it was observed that familial predisposition for atherosclerosis, especially history of coronary artery disease in family members before age

55 (men) and 65 (women) leads to increased cardiovascular risk. It is difficult to separate legacy as an independent factor, especially because other risk factor such as hyperlipoproteinemia, hypertension, coagulation disorders and diabetes have hereditary component. Besides that family can help develop various healthy an unhealthy habits, such as smoking, physical activity, excessive food consumption and obesity, all of which increases the risk of atherosclerosis. It is known that some hereditary lipid disorders of (family hypercholesterolemia, family combined hyperlipidemia), directly cause premature atherosclerosis. Patients with homocystinuria, which is inherited autosomal recessive, usually die from the consequences of atherosclerosis before the age of thirty. If person has a close relative (father, mother or sibling) who has developed CVD before the age of 55, the risk of suffering from a cardiovascular disease is increased two to five fold. The presence of additional risk factors such as high blood pressure, lipid metabolic disorders or diabetes further increases this risk. Families with this particular risk profile require special medical care and preventive measures.

3.2.2 Genotypes and fenotypes

The availability of a wide array of genetic data should also change coronary risk prediction in the future, and many large-scale evaluations of polymorphism and haplotype patterns designed to understand better the atherotrombotic process are well underway. Progress in human genetics holds considerable promise for risk prediction and for individualization of cardiovascular therapy. There are many reports about genes that candidate as predictors of cardiovascular risk. To date, the validation of such genetic markers of risk and drug-responsiveness in multiple populations has often proved disappointing. The advent of technology that permits relatively rapid and inexpensive genome-wide screens and of powerful bioinformatics tools, should spur haplotype analyses and unbiased identification of risk and therapy-response genotypes in the future.

4. Conclusion

There is no doubt that patients with CVD and those with multiple risks factors deserve attention to the term you have particular risk factors extensively and persistently treated. All previous population studies indicate, despite a large palette of new drugs with proven usefulness, many patients who have survived a CVD incident continue smoking, remain overweight, and are treated unsatisfactory. Failure to treat high blood pressure and other risk factors is partly explained by the fact that these patients often simultaneously take several medications with potential side effects. One solution is fixed combination of drugs for treating hypertension, dislipidaemia and diabetes.

CVD prevention refers to all measures taken to prevent their occurrence. It must be carried out in patients who already have documented CVD (coronary disease, previous AMI, stroke, transient ischemic attack, peripheral arteries atherosclerotic disease), hence called the secondary prevention. Primary prevention refers to preventing and treating risk factors in people who have one or more risk factors, but no clinical signs of CVD. Evaluation of the total risk burden is always needed in primary and secondary prevention, and cannot be limited to only one risk factor. Epidemiological studies have proven that many people with an increased risk of CVD, have several risk factors simultaneously, which poses significant challenge to physician.

When it comes to treating dyslipidemia, particularly hypercholesterolemia, all professional societies issued a joint recommendation by which the value of total blood cholesterol should be less than 5.0 mmol/L, and LDL-cholesterol less than 3.0mmol/L. Secondary prevention mandates total cholesterol less than 4.5mmol/L, LDL-cholesterol less than 2,5 mmol/L and blood pressure less than 130/80mmHg, particularly in patients with established CVD, diabetes and renal disease.

Specific focus in prevention is changing of lifestyle habits, solving major cardiovascular risk factors and use of other prophylactic drug therapy for prevention of clinical CVD. All risk factors such as hypertension, adiposity, hypercholesterolemia, diabetes, nicotine use and stress are equally important and present in the development of CVD.

Today, we have a new model to estimate total patients cardiovascular risk - SCORE (Systematic Coronary Risk Evaluation), which is derived from large databases and predicts the total 10-year risk of fatal CVD.

This interactive system of risk assessment aims to provide the physician and patient information on the overall risk and help control interventions. Risk factors, with a completely individual approach to each patient require continuous training complex of the total population in the prevention of risk factors and therefore coronary heart disease.

4.1 Relative risk chart

This chart may used to show younger people at low total risk that, relative to others in their age group, their risk may be many times higher than necessary. This may help to motivate decisions about avoidance of smoking, healthy nutrition and exercise, as well as flagging those who may become candidates for medication (Table 4).

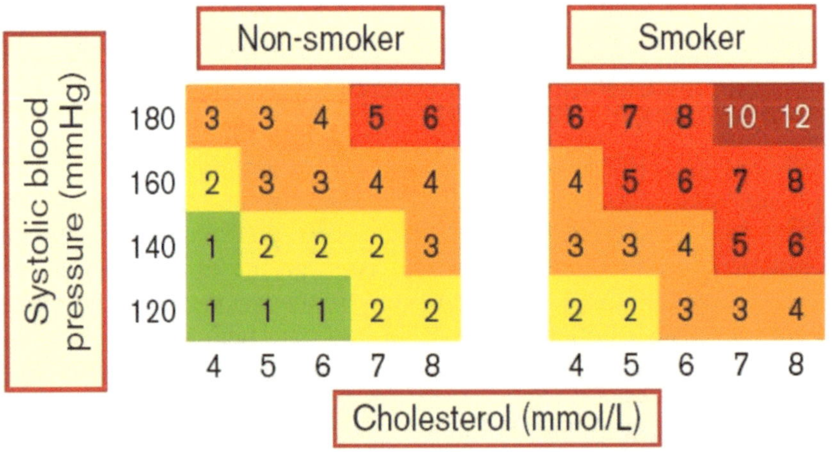

Table 4. Relative risk chart (reproduced from 2004. European guidelines on cardiovascular disease prevention in clinical practice, Croatian Society of Cardiology)

4.2 Stratification of total CV risk

Total CV risk is stratified in four categories. Low, moderate, high and very high risks refer to 10-year risk of fatal or non-fatal CV event. The term „added" indicates that category risk is greater than average. The dashed line indicates how the definition of hypertension (and thus the decision about the initiation of treatment) is flexible, i.e. may be variable depending on the level of total CV risk (Table 4).

Blood pressure (mmHg)					
Other risk factors, OD or Disease	Normal SBP 120-129 or DBP 80-84	High normal SBP 130-139 or DBP 85-89	Grade 1 HT SBP 140-159 or DBP 90-99	Grade 2 HT SBP 160-179 or DBP 100-109	Grade 3 HT SBP≥180 or DBP≥110
No other risk factors	Average risk	Average risk	Low added risk	Moderate added risk	High added risk
1-2 risk factors	Low added risk	Low added risk	Moderate added risk	Moderate added risk	Very high added risk
3 or more risk factors, MS, OD or Diabetes	Moderate added risk	High added risk	High added risk	High added risk	Very high added risk
Established CV or renal disease	Very high added risk	Very high added risk	Very high added risk	Very high added risk	Very high added risk

Table 5. Stratification of CV Risk in four categories. SBP: systolic blood pressure; DBP: diastolic blood pressure; CV: cardiovascular; HT: hypertension. Low,moderate, high and very high risk refer to 10 year risk of a CV fatal or non-fatal event. OD: subclinical organ damage; MS: metabolic syndrome. (Reproduced from 2007.European Guidelines for the management of arterial hypertension, Croatian Society of Hypertension).

Using the SCORE charts, we can assess CVD risk in asymptomatic persons as follows (Table 5, Table 6):

1. use the low risk chart in Belgium, France, Italy, Greece, Luxemburg, Spain, Switzerland and Portugal; use the high risk chart in other countries in Europe
2. Find the cell nearest to the person's age, cholesterol and blood pressure (PB) values, bearing in mind that risk will be higher as the person approaches the next age, cholesterol or BP category
3. Check the qualifiers
4. Establish the total 10-year risk for fatal CVD

Note that a low total cardiovascular risk in a young person may conceal a high relative risk; this may explain to the person by using the relative risk chart. As the person's ages, a high relative risk will translate into a high total risk. More intensive lifestyle advice will need in such persons.

People who stay healthy tend to have certain characteristics:

0 no tobacco
3 walk 3 kilometres daily or 30 minutes any moderate activity
5 portions of fruit and vegetables a day
140 Blood pressure less than 140 systolic
5 total blood cholesterol < 5mmol/L
3 LDL-cholesterol< 3mmol/L
0 avoidance of overweight and diabetes

Continuous training program of the total population in the prevention of risk factors and therefore coronary heart disease, one of the most common causes of morbidity and mortality in developed countries of Europe is mandatory.

Education should start in the younger age groups to prevent the emergence of risk factors, encourage proper diet and lifestyle changes, primarily in the populations who have high total cardiovascular risk. Considering increasing incidence of CVD in rapidly ageing population, prevention is the only way to overcome CVD in the future.

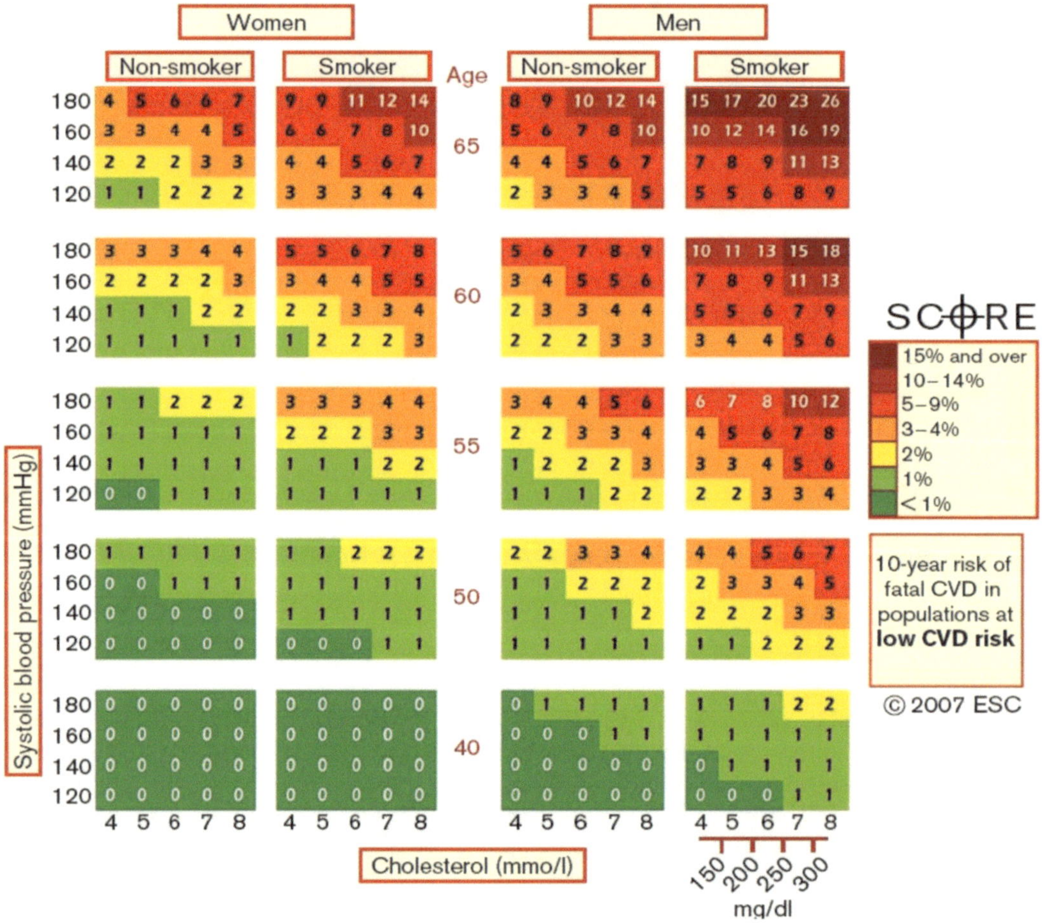

Table 5. 10-year risk of fatal CVD in low risk regions of Europe (reproduced from 2004. European guidelines on cardiovascular disease prevention in clinical practice, Croatian Society of Cardiology)

Age	Systolic blood pressure (mmHg)	Women Non-smoker 4	5	6	7	8	Women Smoker 4	5	6	7	8	Men Non-smoker 4	5	6	7	8	Men Smoker 4	5	6	7	8
65	180	7	8	9	10	12	13	15	17	19	22	14	16	19	22	26	26	30	35	41	47
	160	5	5	6	7	8	9	10	12	13	16	9	11	13	15	16	18	21	25	29	34
	140	3	3	4	5	6	6	7	8	9	11	6	8	9	11	13	13	15	17	20	24
	120	2	2	3	3	4	4	5	5	6	7	4	5	6	7	9	9	10	12	14	17
60	180	4	4	5	6	7	8	9	10	11	13	9	11	13	15	18	18	21	24	28	33
	160	3	3	3	4	5	5	6	7	8	9	6	7	9	10	12	12	14	17	20	24
	140	2	2	2	3	3	3	4	5	5	6	4	5	6	7	9	8	10	12	14	17
	120	1	1	2	2	2	2	3	3	4	4	3	3	4	5	6	6	7	8	10	12
55	180	2	2	3	3	4	4	5	5	6	7	6	7	8	10	12	12	13	16	19	22
	160	1	2	2	2	3	3	3	4	4	5	4	5	6	7	8	8	9	11	13	16
	140	1	1	1	1	2	2	2	2	3	3	3	3	4	5	6	5	6	8	9	11
	120	1	1	1	1	1	1	1	2	2	2	2	2	3	3	4	4	4	5	6	8
50	180	1	1	1	2	2	2	2	3	3	4	4	4	5	6	7	7	8	10	12	14
	160	1	1	1	1	1	1	2	2	2	3	2	3	3	4	5	5	6	7	8	10
	140	0	1	1	1	1	1	1	1	1	2	2	2	2	3	3	3	4	5	6	7
	120	0	0	1	1	1	1	1	1	1	1	1	1	2	2	2	2	3	3	4	5
40	180	0	0	0	0	0	0	0	0	1	1	1	1	1	2	2	2	2	3	3	4
	160	0	0	0	0	0	0	0	0	0	0	1	1	1	1	1	1	2	2	2	3
	140	0	0	0	0	0	0	0	0	0	0	0	1	1	1	1	1	1	1	2	2
	120	0	0	0	0	0	0	0	0	0	0	0	0	1	1	1	1	1	1	1	1

Cholesterol (mmo/l) — 4, 5, 6, 7, 8 (150, 200, 250, 300 mg/dl)

SCORE: 15% and over; 10–14%; 5–9%; 3–4%; 2%; 1%; <1%

10-year risk of fatal CVD in populations at **high CVD risk**

© 2007 ESC

Table 6. 10-year risk of fatal CVD in high-risk regions of Europe (reproduced with permission from 2007. European guidelines on cardiovascular disease prevention in clinical practice, Croatian Society of Cardiology)

5. References

Harrison, T.R. (2008). Harrison' s Principles of Internal medicine, Single edition book, ISBN 978-0-07-159991-7, New York, USA

Ballantyne, C.M.; Keefe, O. Jr. & Gotto, A.M. (2007). Dyslipidemia essentialis, Physican, s Press, ISBN 1-890114-65-0, Michigan, USA

Petrač, D. (2009). Interna medicina, Medicinska naklada, ISBN 978-953-176-391-2, Zagreb, Croatia

McGorrian, C. (2011).Estimating modifiable coronary heart disease risk multiple regions of the world: the INTERHEART Modifiable Risk Score, European Heart Journal, The Zurich Heart House, ISNN 0195-668X; Zurich, Switzerland

Vahanian, A., Ferrari, R. (2010). Compendum of abridged ESC guidelines 2010, Springer Healthcare, ISBN 978-1-907673.9, London, UK.

National Institut of Clinical Excellence (NICE), (August 2004). Clinical Guideline 18, Hypertension: management of hypertension in adults in primary care. NICE London, UK, www.nice.org.uk/CG018NICEguideline.
National Institut of Clinical Exellence (NICE), (March 2010).Quick reference guide, Lipid modification- Cardiovascular risk assessment and modification of blood lipids for the primary and secondary prevention of cardiovascular disease, NICE London, UK,www.niceorg.uk/CG67
Pesek, K. & Pesek, T. (2007). The prevalence of cardiovascular disease risk factor in patient from Croatian Zagorje County treated in Department of Internal medicine General Hospital Zabok from 2000-2006y. Collegium Antropologicum, 31,/Septembar 2007), pp.709-15,ISSN 0350-6134
Pesek, K. & Pesek, T. (2008). Risk Factors Analysis and Diagnoses of Coronary Heart Disease in Patients with Hypercholesterolemia from Croatian Zagorje County, Collegium Antropologicum,32,(April 2008),pp.369-74,ISSN 0350-6134
Hrvatsko kardiološko društvo (HKD), (2004). Europske smjernice za prevenciju bolesti srca i krvnih žila u kliničkoj praksi, Zagreb, Croatia, www.kardio.hr,www.escardio.org
Hvatsko društvo za hipertenziju (HDH), Hrvatsko kardiološko društvo (HKD), (2007). Smjernice za dijagnosticiranje I liječenje arterijske hipertenzije, Zagreb, Croatia, www.kardio.hr www.hdh.hr, www.escardio.org

2

Myocardial Infarction and Angina Pectoris in the History of Medicine on the Polish Soil

Janusz H. Skalski
Jagiellonian University, Cracow
Poland

1. Introduction

This tale concentrates on a fatal affliction that has been permanently associated with human fate since time immemorial, well before *Homo sapiens* were even consciously aware of their existence.

Incidentally, circulatory failure might have developed in the course of various severe diseases, cardiac defects, septic conditions, severe injuries; what is more – it could have been apparent in all age groups. Theoretically, the disease had every chance to have been noted much earlier in the history of mankind than for example ischemic heart disease and the observers might have been our primogenitors-medicians who were blessed with a keen perceptiveness of the rules of nature. Circulatory failure later started to reveal itself only when human life became long enough to allow for natural death to occur, i.e. the demise resulting from biological ageing of the organism could have gained prevalence over the then domineering causes of death: the ever-present homicide in the fight for survival, traumas and infections.

If it comes to that, circulatory failure could be ultimately blamed for natural deaths of the majority of human beings for millions of years. Yet, this is not the point – the point is the history of rational recognizing and well thought-out attempts at treating the disease that in its nature is the expression of an upset balance of the circulatory system. Here we need to assume that in the history of medicine, the form of circulatory failure being a consequence of non-cardiac diseases, or in other words a simple circulatory complication of another, inevitably fatal disease, could not have been differentiated by ancient physicians from primary ailments of the cardiovascular system.

In the practice of a historian of medicine, it is much simpler to pick out from historical tests information on the terminal stage of – say - coronary heart disease with its drastic incidents of pain than to find reports on mundane deterioration of health, gradual waning of life amidst not quite spectacular symptoms (with some exceptions, though) that were treated as a natural end of life. It is worthwhile, then, to start with such evident descriptions of a severe heart disease, where we also can find properties pointing to circulatory failure. Indeed, the very *circulatory failure* as an ailment with which ancient physicians could not successfully cope, always had to end with the demise of a patient that was treated as the so-called "natural death".

Throughout the period when - through partitions - Poland was robbed of existing as an independent nation, in the years 1795-1918, the Polish soil became the home country of numerous illustrious Europeans of various nationalities; here, the history of medicine was developed not only by native Polish nationals. We should remember about their ties with the country, which - by choice or by chance - become their home. In this context, the present paper describes Silesians – Bishop Thomas of Wrocław or A.Ch. Thebesius - in the case of which there are no grounds to count them as members of the Polish society.

On the other hand, Polish scientists who made great contribution to the development of world medicine in the 19th century, but had no home country, were often customarily treated as nationals of the occupant countries. Many of those scientists form a group of obscure research workers– unknown to the public at large not only due to lack of national separateness lasting for more than a century (e.g. Józef Chrzczonowicz, Jan Cenner, Andrzej Janikowski, Józef Rompalski, Napoleon Cybulski, etc.), but also because they most commonly described their achievements in the Polish language, unknown to the universal milieu of great scientists and discoverers (Józef Pawiński, Władysław Biegański, Walery Jaworski, Józef Latkowski, etc.). The times have changed, but recalling the nationality of those individuals and at the same time, their contribution to the development of medicine is our duty, although we live in a different reality, in the common and peaceful Europe that unites many nations and respects national differences. The above arguments justify recalling the history of *angina pectoris* in a central-eastern European country, since scientists who lived there years ago deserve to be remembered.

2. Polish medicine in the Middle Ages

It is impossible to discuss the history of understanding and treating coronary heart disease and myocardial infarction in Poland in separation from the ancient history of world medicine – the former was a part of the latter, albeit very small, although it had a chance of existing on the Polish soil only in the Middle Ages.

We know well that the oldest inscriptions, the content of which may be related to symptoms of coronary heart disease were found as early as in ancient Egyptian papyruses written approximately 3500 ago, in notes from the Middle or Far East, shrouded in mysticism, prejudice and scientific helplessness, or in the legacy of the Mediterranean medicine. We are not certain as to the character of the described ailments; we do not know whether the authors were indeed writing about the signs of angina pectoris and myocardial infarction.

Hydrops, undoubtedly associated with circulatory failure, cardiac disease and – indirectly – also with coronary disease and its consequences, was treated since the ancient times (Egypt, Greece) with sea onion *(Urginea maritima)*. In the Middle Ages, in central and eastern Europe, lily-of-the valley *(Convallaria majalis)* was used to achieve the same purpose. With the exception of these examples, in those times, we will not find any more interesting descriptions of therapeutic concepts that might refer to heart diseases. In the dark and scholastic Middle Ages or even at the time when Renaissance sciences flourished, we still see no progress. With respect to diagnosing and understanding the nature of heart diseases, the situation was similar if not grimmer. Only the turn of the 16th and 17th centuries did bring some break-through.

Along with the considerably dubious progress of medicine in the Middle Ages, medical thought was slowly and timidly developing in Poland as well. As in the entire European medicine of those times – although with infrequent exceptions – also in Poland there was not a single attempt made at searching for a cause of death resulting from heart ailments.

Possibly only the text on heart diseases included in a fairly well known in Medieval Europe manuscript entitled *Practica Medicinalis,* which was written on the Polish soil, is worth mentioning as an exception in the medicine of the Middle Ages. Its author was Thomas of Wrocław, the Titular Bishop of Sarepta.

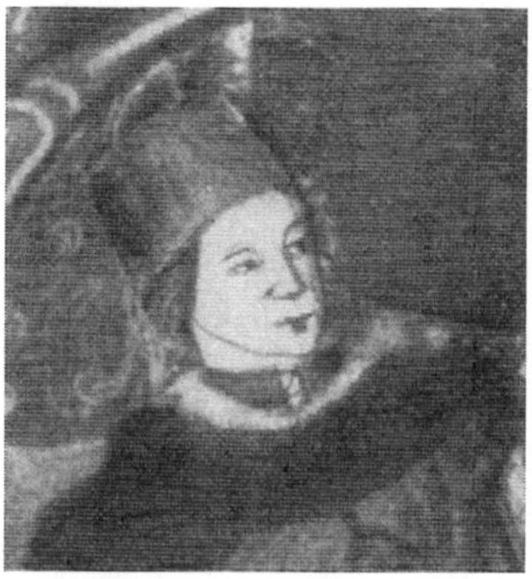

Fig. 1. Bishop Thomas of Wrocław (1297 - ca. 1378)

Most likely, he came from Silesia, studied medical sciences in Montpellier, Salerno, Padua, and Bologna, and was well-travelled. Later, already as a well-acclaimed scientist, he was invited as a lecturer to the universities of Paris, Montpellier and Oxford. He was a physician to Pope John XXII, Prince Henryk IV and Czech kings: John of Luxembourg and Charles IV (Skalski & Stembrowicz, 2004). The history of cardiology and the works of Bishop Thomas are associated through one of 202 chapters of this manuscript entitled *De syncopi et debilitate cordis* – the text discusses "disability"([1]) of the heart, palpitations and the resultant syncope. This was the first Polish dissertation referring to the heart and possibly the first work worldwide that observed an association between loss of consciousness and disturbances in cardiac action. We are not certain what is meant by some sentences. To give an example: "...there appears a malevolent attribute of cold, horrible for the heart (...). This is supported by the heart's weakness, while its movement is turned into torment. And thus, disability of the heart ensues promptly. And when indeed a fainting spell is prolonged and movement and sensation in the body are lost, death occurs most frequently" (Stembrowicz, 1994).

A lot is left to the imagination of the reader, as well as to the translation of the convoluted and highly scholastic text, abounding in philosophical adornments. In free translation and interpretation, the above quoted fragment might be easily regarded a description of a severe heart disease...

In the 16th century Poland, the level of medical sciences - represented solely in Krakow - was relatively low. Here, the physiological interpretations of Hippocrates, Galen and Avicenna were still upheld. Nevertheless, we could risk speaking about the beginnings of a genuine Polish interest in anatomy and physiology. Numerous works were written by native authors, where they demonstrated associations between the heart and vascular system. Among them, a treatise of obstetrics by Piotr Cziachowski (1620) should be mentioned, with its chapter on *Heart beating and fainting spells in the pregnant*. The chapter contains a fragment, where the author – somewhat clumsily – attempts to explain the cause of weakness and fainting spells by cardiac dysfunction.

---

[1] „debilitas" may be translated as weakness, feebleness, insufficient function, debilitation, or – in a completely free translation – disease.

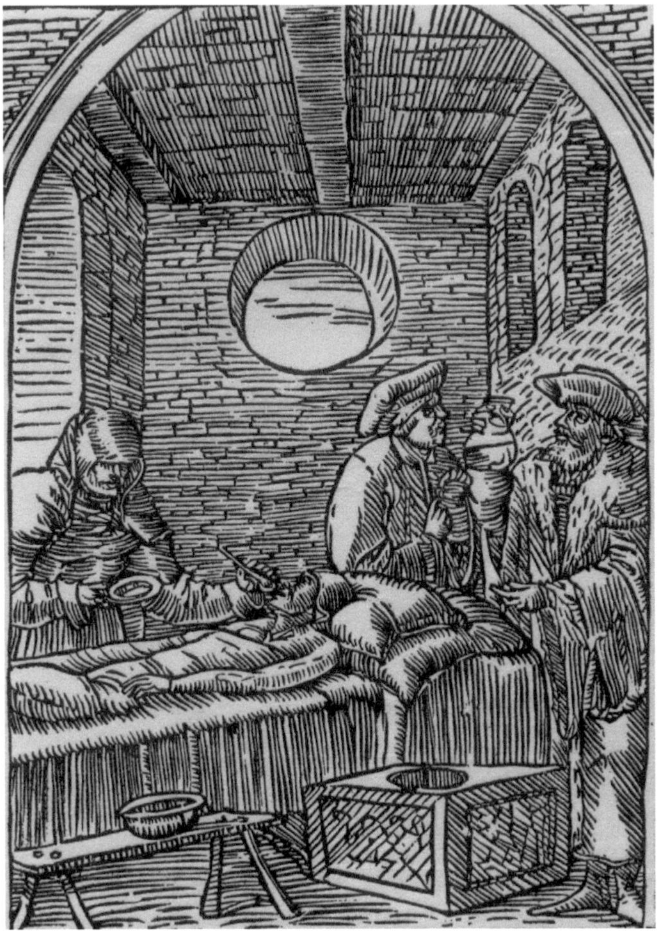

Fig. 2. Case consultation for a severely ill patient. Armorial published in Krakow, 1568 (authored by Marcin Siennik).

Many a century has passed since Aulus Cornelius Celsus (53 B. C. - 7 A.D.), a scientist, naturalist and encyclopedist and a considerable Roman intellectualist, drew attention to a prognostic importance of edemas, thus becoming the discoverer of water balance disturbances. For the sake of understanding circulatory failure, we should remember that the works of Celsus most likely contain the first accurate diagnostic indication, medical order and an attempt at establishing a diagnosis, all of them previously unheard of. Namely, in a patient with hydrops, he recommended: ..."one should cautiously measure the belly using a thread and in this way pay attention to its size; thus, one sees whether the belly is more or less extended. If the belly is smaller, it means the medications acted beneficially. One should also calculate the amount of fluids given to the patient and the amount of urine he passes. If the patient passes more urine than the volume of fluids he drinks, one may hope for his recovery".

Only in the 16th and 17th centuries did physicians again take interest in edemas and hydrops; many a decade had to pass until in the 18th century, they slowly started to also perceive an association between the above signs and cardiac dysfunction, although the cause of hydrops could be indeed diversified. In this respect we also should mention a work by a Polish author, Jan Innocenty Petrycy - *De hydrope,* based on which he sought incorporation to the Krakow Academy, which was effected on April 2, 1620. This interesting dissertation has become a part of the world medical literature as one of the first reports in this field (Skalski, 2009).

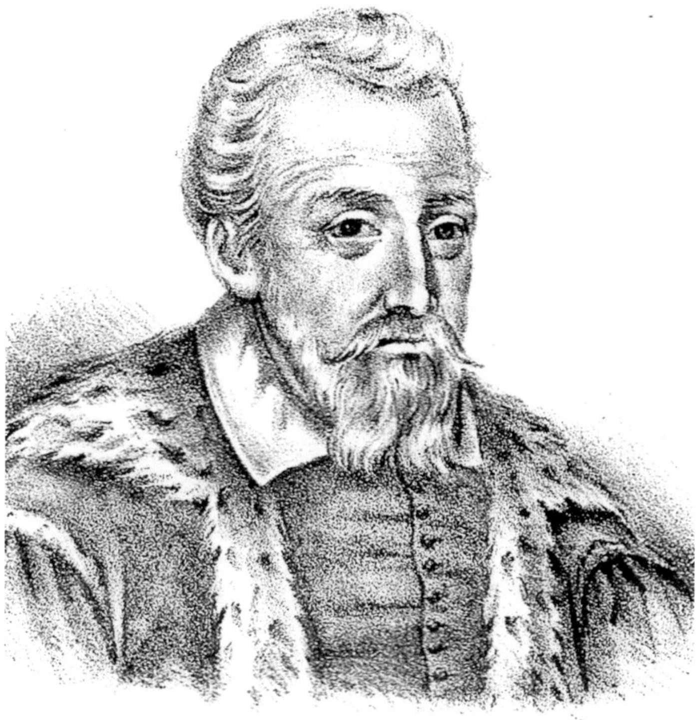

Fig. 3. Jan Innocenty Petrycy (?-†1641)

In keeping with the rules of the then practiced medicine, in case of hydrops, to eliminate edemas, abdominal puncture and drainage were recommended. For three consecutive centuries, this was a commonly employed method of – as we would say today – symptomatic treatment of the effects of circulatory failure, and thus also of severe coronary disease. The method somewhat lost its relevance when digitalis was introduced at the end of the 18th century, but it persevered in the 19th century, and in a modernized form - until the contemporary times.

Chest pain was still associated with a mysterious and malevolent disease of unknown etiology. No one could pinpoint the source of pain and ascertain whether it originated in the respiratory tract, lungs, heart, vessels, esophagus or the cardia. And the patient, with his unskilled and naïve accounts, could not provide any leading clues to the embarrassed and oftentimes opinionated physician, since there was a common lack of understanding of the nature of such ailments. After all, in Latin, the term "*cardia*" denotes the part of the stomach attached to the esophagus... In 18th and 19th-century dictionaries, "*cardiacus*" means either "cordial" or a remedy against ailments involving the heart and stomach, while pain felt in this area is termed "*cardialgia*" (Richter, 1671).

3. The discovery of coronary artery disease and myocardial infarction

Many of my Colleagues who are reading this chapter now may find unbelievable that in this central and eastern part of Europe, most likely for the first time ever in the history of medicine, atherosclerotic lesions involving the coronary arteries, possibly a direct cause of death of the autopsied patient, were observed. A physician who made such an observation was Adam Christian Thebesius, who described - if not the first, then surely as one among the first physicians - "ossification" of coronary arteries. This was the term he used then to denote coronary arteriosclerosis. Although he did not use the Polish language, was German, and - to be more precise - his home country was simply Silesia, where he spent almost his entire life and worked, I am mentioning his name with a degree of satisfaction, recalling his ties with the Polish soil.

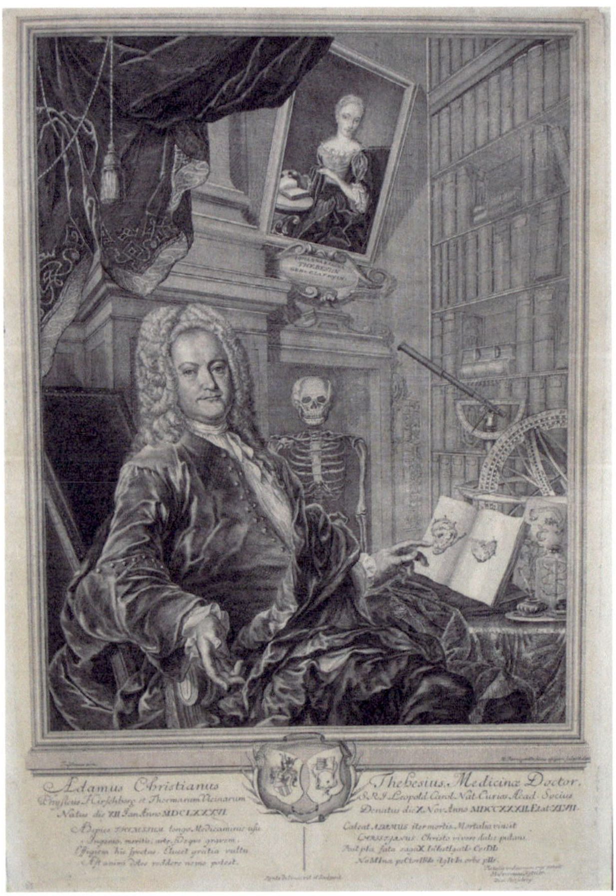

Fig. 4. Adam Christian Thebesius (1686-1732)

Thebesius was one of the most eminent students of heart anatomy, in particular a pioneer of studies on coronary circulation, an expert in the anatomy of coronary vessels and the first to describe their anomalies. Such terms as the "Thebesian veins" and the "valve of Thebesius" are commonly known in the anatomical nomenclature of the heart and recognized in the entire contemporary medical world.

Born in Lower Silesia, Thebesius studied in Leipzig, Halle and Leiden. When 22 years old, in 1708, in Leiden, he was conferred the title of doctor of medical sciences based on his innovative dissertation on coronary circulation entitled *Disputatio medica inauguralis de circulo sanquinis in corde.* Having intentionally given up all his university positions and honors, he settled in Jelenia Gora. Six years later, in 1714, he was entrusted with an honorable position of a "city physicist" (an equivalent of a municipal physician), which he held for 20 years. He died at the age of 47 years due to pneumonia that developed in the course of asthma (Domosławski, 1967, Skalski & Kuch, 2006).

An eminent place in development of the history of ischemic heart disease is occupied by Giovanni B. Morgagni (1682-1771), the founder of clinical anatomopathology. Morgagni searched for and managed to find lesions involving various organs that were the cause of a disease or death. In 1761, he published a splendid work consisting of letters-articles, mostly case reports, entitled *De sedibus et causis morborum per anatomen indagatis libri quinque,* or, in other words, five volumes focusing on location and putative caused of diseases. In some of Morgagni's "letters" we can easily find descriptions of angina pectoris. In a woman who died presenting with chest pain and dyspnea, he described in the autopsy protocol numerous ossifications involving the aorta and arteries branching off from the aorta.

The knowledge of anatomy of the coronary vessels and the observation of pathological lesions, even when they were encountered incidentally, in a natural way inspired physicians to searching for causative associations between the observed lesions and intravital clinical signs, especially with chest pain. However, in the 18th century, the knowledge of coronary vessel anatomy reached a relatively high level. At long last, there came the time for a genuine "discovery" of ischemic heart disease and myocardial infarction. The discovery of a "new or hitherto unknown disease", as it was referred to, crystallized into certainty; its authors were two physicians, who independently published their observations in 1768: Nicolas Rougnon de Magny (1727-1799), a physician from France, and William Heberden (1710-1801) - a British doctor. The discovery was of a grave importance. Although it was Rougnon who used in his report the strongly put term "a hitherto unknown disease" to describe coronary disease, yet it was not Rougnon, but Heberden who was and is still associated with the "discovery" and for long years to come, as late as in the 19th century, the condition was called "Heberden's disease" (Willius & Dry, 1948).

On July 21, 1768, Heberden presented his memorable lecture during a meeting of the Royal College of Physicians in London entitled *Some account of a disorder of the breast.* In addition to a fairly accurate presentation of the course of the disease and the character of complaints, the paper described the helplessness of a physician with respect to possible treatment, presenting a pessimistic attitude and a sense of resignation. (Pawiński, 1908; Willius&Dry, 1948; Stembrowicz, 1987)

4. "Angina pectoris" in the oldest Polish literature

For the subsequent several score years, in the atmosphere of therapeutic nihilism and - to put it mildly - lack of optimism as to the proposed treatment, in various parts of Europe, and obviously also in Poland, there appeared scientific reports. Within a few years, the new disease entity was accepted by the medical world, what is not tantamount to all physicians acknowledging it without a grain of salt (Ruciński&Skalski 2004). The then concept of a patient suffering from some general "chest breathlessness" was too deeply rooted, and the very "breathlessness" was understood in a different way, oftentimes based on prejudice, fanciful diagnoses that today evoke a snicker of tolerant irony.

On the Polish soil, the harbingers of recognizing *angina pectoris* appeared relatively early, but obviously not immediately. In this very spirit a young physician from Vilnius Józef Chrzczonowicz (1790-1823) wrote in 1812 his doctoral dissertation entitled *Dissertatio inauguralis medica de angore pectoris* (2). Chrzczonowicz, a student of Józef Frank (1771-1842), himself an eminent and well-educated clinician, described in his thesis not only the signs of the disease, but also autopsy results of patients who died of angina pectoris. Chrzczonowicz was a very young physician when he submitted his doctoral dissertation, he was only 22 years old and had received a diploma only two years before (Chrzczonowicz, 1812).
Referring to W. Heberden and J. Forthergill, he reported that during autopsies one could observe ossification of the heart, coronary arteries, aorta and semilunar valves; incidentally, most likely he himself neither performed postmortem examinations not participated in autopsies. Against all common beliefs, he stated that the disease was rather common, mostly affected elderly males, was less often encountered in females and seen mostly in postmenstrual women. The author of the dissertation performed a differential diagnosis of four - in his opinion easily mistaken - conditions: angina pectoris, "periodic breathlessness" [author's note - bronchial asthma], nightmare (!) and fainting spells. Among numerous clinical observations, his descriptions of pain reported by the patients are the most accurate: "pain situated in the lower sternum, extending to the back, ears and through the upper extremities, sometimes involving the hand".
Eight years later, a doctoral dissertation with a title similar to that used by Chrzczonowicz was submitted by a young Cracovian physician Jan Cenner. The doctoral exam open to the public took place in the Jagiellonian University on July 14, 1820 (Chrzczonowicz, 1812; Cenner, 1820).
Cenner lacked support of an experienced supervisor and thus his situation was much worse than that of his older colleague from Vilnius, Chrzczonowicz. Undoubtedly, the supervisor of the latter, the above mentioned Józef Frank, could have much more effectively helped the candidate for doctor's degree both by shaping the idea underlining the dissertation and by his professional expertise. The Krakow university was somewhat behind the Vilnius school, and the professors working with Cenner were unquestionably less experienced in recognizing and treating heart diseases.
In the work of Cenner, similarly as in the case of Chrzczonowicz, the majority of what could be deemed novel was transferred from the cited bibliographical items. Even so, the dissertation prepared by Cenner seems to be an almost encyclopedic listing of medical knowledge on angina pectoris in the early 19th century (Śliwiński, 1976).
Cenner reported as a reliable and verified piece of information that autopsies performed in patients with angina pectoris demonstrated "calcification" of the coronary vessels, walls of large arteries and heart valves. Yet, while reading his text, we have an impression that the said ossification of vessels is treated as a curiosity rather than a sign of the principal nature of the disease. Some of the proposed medical measures seem today bizarre and incomprehensible, others have some deeper meaning, since through a cascade of physiological phenomena they triggered they might have helped the patient to some degree. Our attention is drawn to the use of digitalis and opium. In addition, Cenner's dissertation discussed numerous therapeutic measures, the use of which seems justified today and testifies to a brilliant intuition of physicians practicing the profession at that time. To use some examples, recommendations proposed in those days included snakeroot

[2] the Latin term „angor" denotes both suffocation, breathlessness, anxiety and fear.

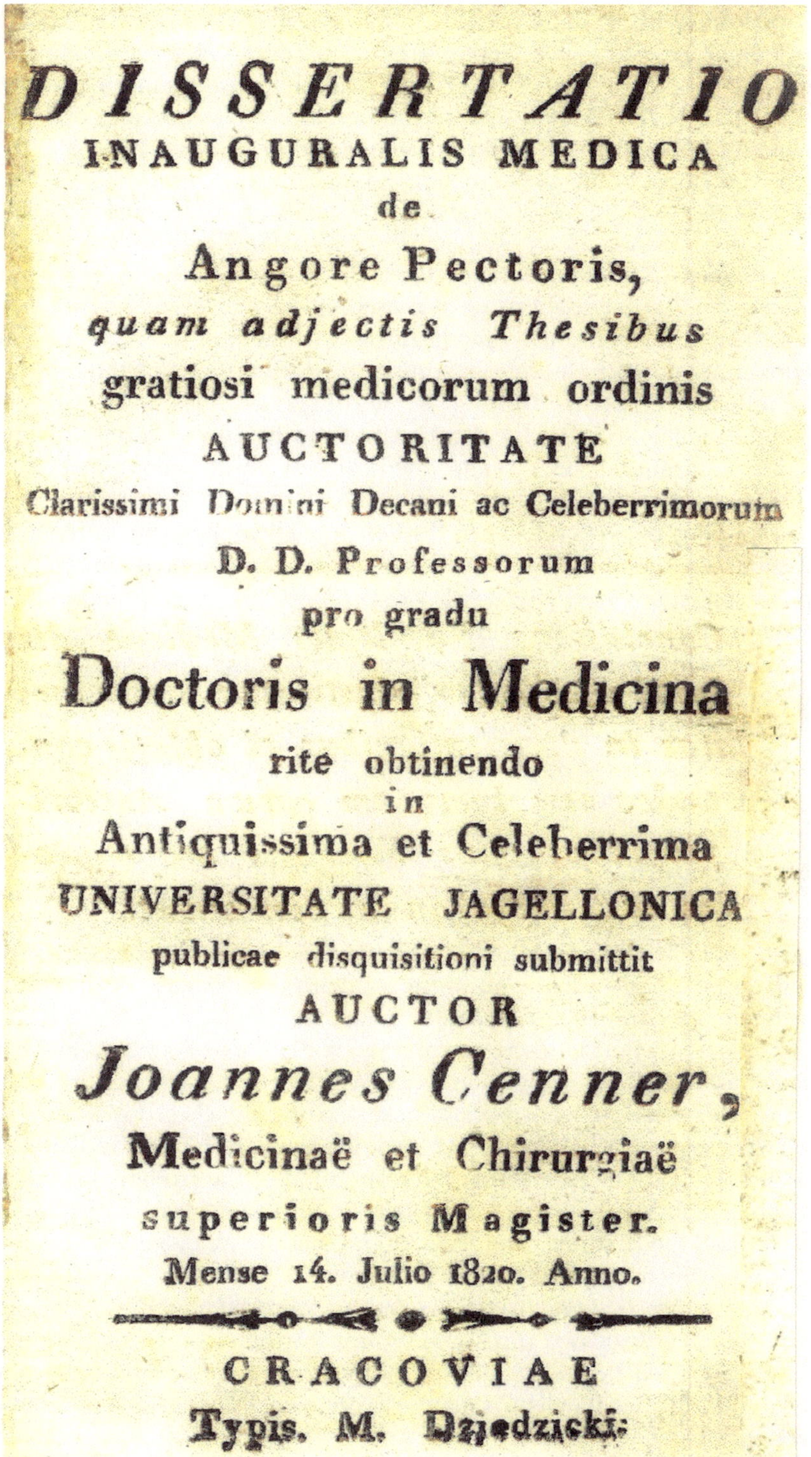

DISSERTATIO
INAUGURALIS MEDICA
de
Angore Pectoris,
quam adjectis Thesibus
gratiosi medicorum ordinis
AUCTORITATE
Clarissimi Domini Decani ac Celeberrimorum
D. D. Professorum
pro gradu
Doctoris in Medicina
rite obtinendo
in
Antiquissima et Celeberrima
UNIVERSITATE JAGELLONICA
publicae disquisitioni submittit
AUCTOR
Joannes Cenner,
Medicinaë et Chirurgiaë
superioris Magister.
Mense 14. Julio 1820. Anno.

CRACOVIAE
Typis. M. Dziedzicki.

Fig. 5. The title page of Jan Cenner's doctoral dissertation entitled "De angore pectoris".

(*Rauvolfia serpentyna,* with its anti-arrhythmic, hypotensive and anxiolytic effects), angelica (a spasmolytic and diuretic agent, today known to contain a calcium channel blocker), magnesium salts (anti-arrhythmic), potassium carbonate (a donor of potassium ions), Peruvian cinchona bark (its alkaloids quinine and quinidine show an anti-arrhythmic effect), henbane bell (a relaxant effect, e.g. in bronchial asthma) or calcium carbonate (as a donor of calcium ions). In contrast to the above mentioned medications, numerous agents are simply bizarre and their use may be today regarded erroneous and irrational, since they include poisons posing the patient's life at risk, such as copper and gold salts, calomel, cinnabar, hemlock, laurel water (it contains an ingredient that is degraded into hydrogen cyanide!); some irritating agents for external use are also unfounded.

Still others represent long-forgotten medications with anxiolytic, relaxing and analgesic properties (musk, castoreum, asafetida, stink lettuce, leaf stems of bittersweet, etc.) and dehydrating effects. What is striking in addition to numerous recommendations associated with hygiene and diet, is attention to fluid balance ("large amounts of fluids, tea, coffee are contraindicated...") and medical advice to avoid alcohol and other condiments (Skalski et al., 2003).

The problem of angina pectoris returns in the Polish medical literature only after another 24 years, and thus we see that the subject was not then counted among issues being particularly fashionable. A rather interesting case report by Andrzej Janikowski, Chairman of the Warsaw Medical Society, described *angina pectoris* diagnosed intravitally in a patient, in whom the antemortal diagnosis was confirmed on autopsy. Janikowski's article entitled "Ossification of coronary arteries of the heart", although short, is, nevertheless, the first Polish report based on modern scientific pragmatism and at the same time written in keeping with the principles of clinical pathology, with a postmortem confirmation of the diagnosis (Janikowski, 1844).

4. The lifetime diagnosis of the myocardial infaction

In 1850, the Tygodnik Lekarski [the Medical Weekly] published a paper by Józef Rompalski on angina pectoris ("Heberden's asthma, *angina pectoris, stenocardia, etc."*), where the author described a death of a patient who had presented with unmistakable signs that might have resulted solely from a completed myocardial infarction. Thus, we acknowledge the report by Rompalski as the first Polish description of myocardial infarction, despite the fact that the patient was not autopsied. The paper is in its entirety based on a case report describing a 69-year old male who suffered from periodic chest pain and chest 'squeezing' "below the sternal bone". The pain was explosive and crushing in character and radiated through the left neck to the left shoulder and elbow; the respiration of the patient was "depressed and restless". Another episode, which occurred two months later, lasted 15 minutes and was more intensive than the first one. The third, 30-minute attack preceded a series of rapidly repeated episodes, which the patient failed to survive.

Based on the reported case, Rompalski presented his knowledge of the causes of the disease he was aware of: "The discussed disease is typical for the second half of human lifespan, being rarely encountered before the 40th or 50th year of age (...) amidst the most prettily blooming health, it terrifies its victims. Its duration is very changeable and the end almost always fatal (...). Almost at all times, more or less complete ossifications are found involving the coronary arteries, along with injuries of the aorta, thickening, ulcerations and calcifications of this great artery" (Skalski, 2004).

A whole century had passed since the publication of the landmark paper by William Heberden on angina pectoris until myocardial infarction as its most severe complication was diagnosed in a living patient based on clinical presentation.

The first such intravital diagnosis was established by an Austrian physician Adam Hammer (1818-1878) in 1878. He described a case of a coronary embolism in a 34-year old male diagnosed when the patient was alive and subsequently confirmed by autopsy. The patient died manifesting signs of cardiogenic shock, pronounced bradycardia, but immediately before death, he did not complain of stenocardiac pain. The autopsy demonstrated a complete occlusion of the left coronary artery ostium caused by a thrombus, which filled the entire right coronary sinus of Valsalva (Lie, 1978).

Nine years later (1887), a Polish physician, a phenomenal clinician and a great scientist, Professor Edward Sas-Korczyński published in Krakow a paper aptly entitled "Coronary artery embolism (*Embolia arteriae coronariae cordis*) diagnosed in a living patient". The report discussed a clinical course similar to that observed by his Austrian predecessor. Unfortunately, the article by Korczyński, published in his native language, remained virtually unknown in the world and was rarely quoted in the literature worldwide. A pity, though, since the unique character of the observations, extraordinary scientific inquisitiveness, conscientious clinical description (the total number of pages in the report equaled 9) and finally, a thoughtfully selected bibliography place the work of Korczyński among the most important clinical reports in the world of the 19th century (Korczyński, 1887; Pamiętniki Jubileuszowy..., 1900).

The report by Korczyński, predominantly based on clinical aspects, had preceded a publication dated 1910 and authored by W. P. Obrastzow and N. D. Straschesko of Kiev, which - as it should be truthfully said - provided a precise description of a clinical presentation of a coronary embolus (myocardial infarction) and for this reason is believed to represent a break-through in the field (Obrastzow & Staschesko, 1910).

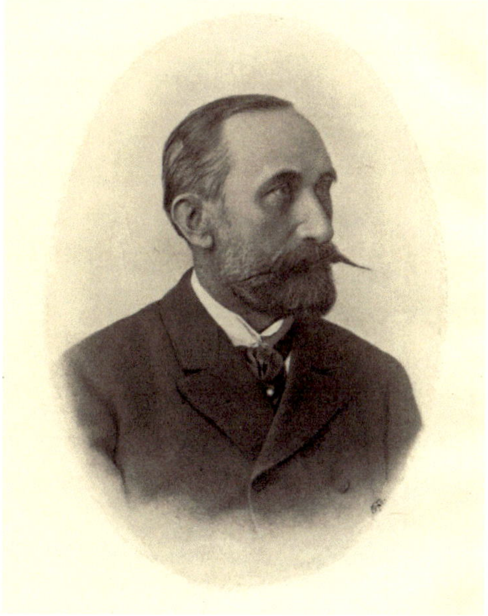

Fig. 6. Edward Sas-Korczyński (1844-1905)

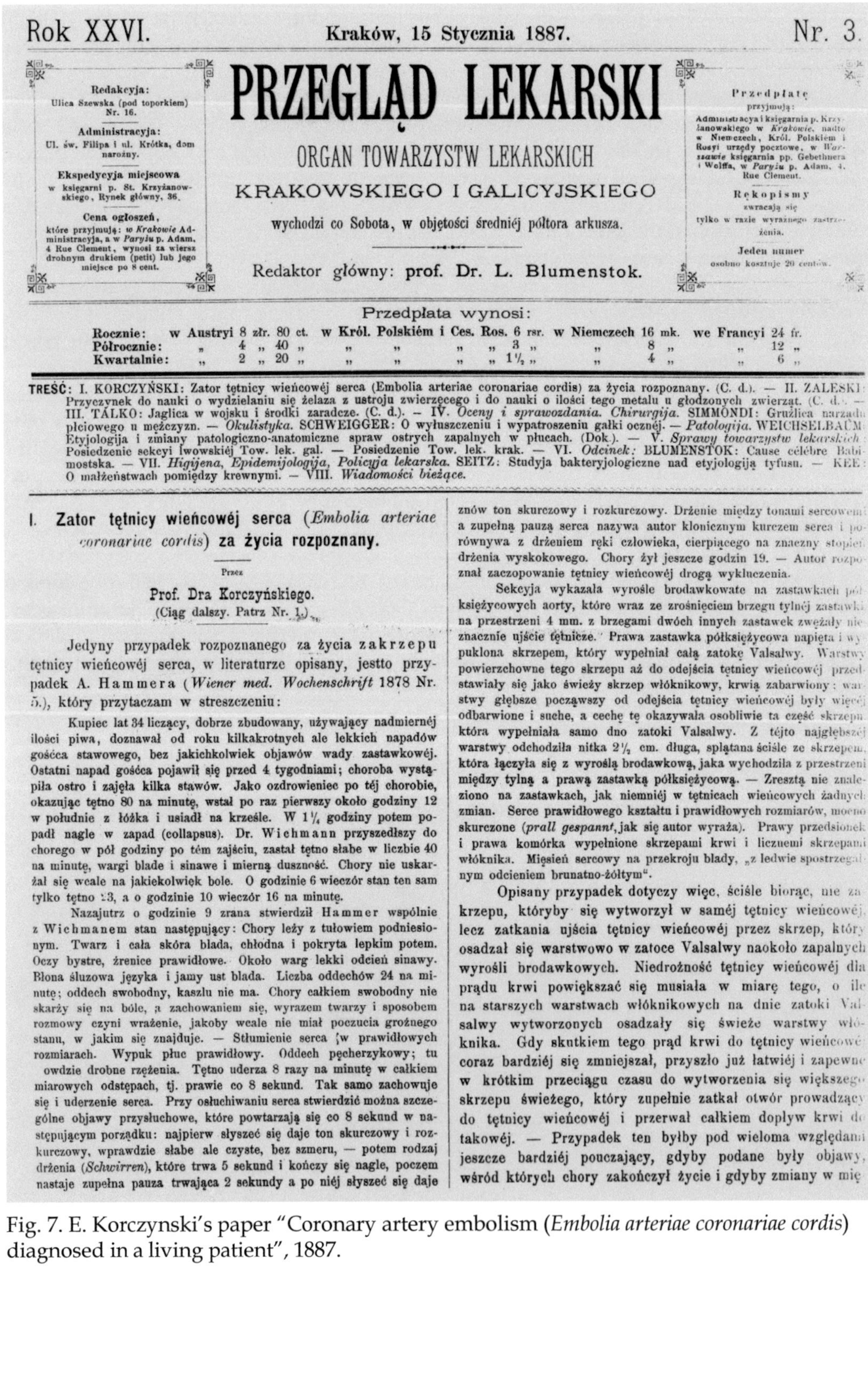

Rok XXVI. Kraków, 15 Stycznia 1887. Nr. 3.

PRZEGLĄD LEKARSKI

ORGAN TOWARZYSTW LEKARSKICH

KRAKOWSKIEGO I GALICYJSKIEGO

wychodzi co Sobota, w objętości średniéj półtora arkusza.

Redaktor główny: prof. Dr. L. Blumenstok.

Redakcyja: Ulica Szewska (pod toporkiem) Nr. 16.

Administracyja: Ul. św. Filipa i ul. Krótka, dom narożny.

Ekspedycyja miejscowa w księgarni p. St. Krzyżanowskiego, Rynek główny, 36.

Cena ogłoszeń, które przyjmują: *w Krakowie* Administracyja, a w *Paryżu* p. Adam, 4 Rue Clement, wynosi za wiersz drobnym drukiem (petit) lub jego miejsce po 8 cent.

Przedpłatę przyjmują: Administracya i księgarnia p. Krzyżanowskiego w *Krakowie*, nadto w Niemczech, Król. Polskiém i Rosyi urzędy pocztowe, w *Warszawie* księgarnia pp. Gebethnera i Wolffa, w *Paryżu* p. Adam, 4, Rue Clement.

Rękopismy zwracają się tylko w razie wyraźnego zastrzeżenia.

Jeden numer osobno kosztuje 20 centów.

Przedpłata wynosi:

Rocznie:	w Austryi 8 złr. 80 ct.	w Król. Polskiém i Ces. Ros. 6 rsr.	w Niemczech 16 mk.	we Francyi 24 fr.
Półrocznie:	„ 4 „ 40 „	„ „ „ „ 3 „	„ 8 „	„ 12 „
Kwartalnie:	„ 2 „ 20 „	„ „ „ „ 1½ „	„ 4 „	„ 6 „

I. Zator tętnicy wieńcowéj serca (*Embolia arteriae coronariae cordis*) za życia rozpoznany.

Przez

Prof. Dra Korczyńskiego.

(Ciąg dalszy. Patrz Nr. 1.)

Jedyny przypadek rozpoznanego za życia zakrzepu tętnicy wieńcowéj serca, w literaturze opisany, jestto przypadek A. Hammera (*Wiener med. Wochenschrift* 1878 Nr. 5.), który przytaczam w streszczeniu:

Kupiec lat 34 liczący, dobrze zbudowany, używający nadmiernéj ilości piwa, doznawał od roku kilkakrotnych ale lekkich napadów gośćca stawowego, bez jakichkolwiek objawów wady zastawkowéj. Ostatni napad gośćca pojawił się przed 4 tygodniami; choroba wystąpiła ostro i zajęła kilka stawów. Jako ozdrowieniec po téj chorobie, okazując tętno 80 na minutę, wstał po raz pierwszy około godziny 12 w południe z łóżka i usiadł na krześle. W 1¼ godziny potem popadł nagle w zapad (collapsus). Dr. Wichmann przyszedłszy do chorego w pół godziny po tém zajściu, zastał tętno słabe w liczbie 40 na minutę, wargi blade i sinawe i mierną duszność. Chory nie uskarżał się wcale na jakiekolwiek bole. O godzinie 6 wieczór stan ten sam tylko tętno 23, a o godzinie 10 wieczór 16 na minutę.

Nazajutrz o godzinie 9 zrana stwierdził Hammer wspólnie z Wichmanem stan następujący: Chory leży z tułowiem podniesionym. Twarz i cała skóra blada, chłodna i pokryta lepkim potem. Oczy bystre, źrenice prawidłowe. Około warg lekki odcień sinawy. Błona śluzowa języka i jamy ust blada. Liczba oddechów 24 na minutę; oddech swobodny, kaszlu nie ma. Chory całkiem swobodny nie skarży się na bóle, a zachowaniem się, wyrazem twarzy i sposobem rozmowy czyni wrażenie, jakoby wcale nie miał poczucia groźnego stanu, w jakim się znajduje. — Stłumienie serca w prawidłowych rozmiarach. Wypuk płuc prawidłowy. Oddech pęcherzykowy; tu owdzie drobne rzężenia. Tętno uderza 8 razy na minutę w całkiem miarowych odstępach, tj. prawie co 8 sekund. Tak samo zachowuje się i uderzenie serca. Przy osłuchiwaniu serca stwierdzić można szczególne objawy przysłuchowe, które powtarzają się co 8 sekund w następującym porządku: najpierw słyszeć się daje ton skurczowy i rozkurczowy, wprawdzie słabe ale czyste, bez szmeru, — potem rodzaj drżenia (*Schwirren*), które trwa 5 sekund i kończy się nagle, poczem nastaje zupełna pauza trwająca 2 sekundy a po niéj słyszeć się daje znów ton skurczowy i rozkurczowy. Drżenie między tonami sercowemi a zupełną pauzą serca nazywa autor klonicznym kurczem serca i porównywa z drżeniem ręki człowieka, cierpiącego na znaczny stopień drżenia wyskokowego. Chory żył jeszcze godzin 19. — Autor rozpoznał zaczopowanie tętnicy wieńcowéj drogą wykluczenia.

Sekcyja wykazała wyrośle brodawkowate na zastawkach półksiężycowych aorty, które wraz ze zrośnięciem brzegu tylnéj zastawki na przestrzeni 4 mm. z brzegami dwóch innych zastawek zwężały nieznacznie ujście tętnicze. Prawa zastawka półksiężycowa napięta i wypuklona skrzepem, który wypełniał całą zatokę Valsalwy. Warstwy powierzchowne tego skrzepu aż do odejścia tętnicy wieńcowéj przedstawiały się jako świeży skrzep włóknikowy, krwią zabarwiony; warstwy głębsze począwszy od odejścia tętnicy wieńcowéj były więcéj odbarwione i suche, a cechę tę okazywała osobliwie ta część skrzepu która wypełniała samo dno zatoki Valsalwy. Z téjto najgłębszéj warstwy odchodziła nitka 2½ cm. długa, splątana ściśle ze skrzepem, która łączyła się z wyroślą brodawkową, jaka wychodziła z przestrzeni między tylną a prawą zastawką półksiężycową. — Zresztą nie znaleziono na zastawkach, jak niemniéj w tętnicach wieńcowych żadnych zmian. Serce prawidłowego kształtu i prawidłowych rozmiarów, mocno skurczone (*prall gespannt*, jak się autor wyraża). Prawy przedsionek i prawa komórka wypełnione skrzepami krwi i licznemi skrzepami włóknika. Mięsień sercowy na przekroju blady, „z ledwie spostrzegalnym odcieniem brunatno-żółtym".

Opisany przypadek dotyczy więc, ściśle biorąc, nie zakrzepu, któryby się wytworzył w saméj tętnicy wieńcowéj, lecz zatkania ujścia tętnicy wieńcowéj przez skrzep, który osadzał się warstwowo w zatoce Valsalwy naokoło zapalnych wyrośli brodawkowych. Niedrożność tętnicy wieńcowéj dla prądu krwi powiększać się musiała w miarę tego, o ile na starszych warstwach włóknikowych na dnie zatoki Valsalwy wytworzonych osadzały się świeże warstwy włóknika. Gdy skutkiem tego prąd krwi do tętnicy wieńcowéj coraz bardziéj się zmniejszał, przyszło już łatwiéj i zapewne w krótkim przeciągu czasu do wytworzenia się większego skrzepu świeżego, który zupełnie zatkał otwór prowadzący do tętnicy wieńcowéj i przerwał całkiem dopływ krwi do takowéj. — Przypadek ten byłby pod wieloma względami jeszcze bardziéj pouczający, gdyby podane były objawy, wśród których chory zakończył życie i gdyby zmiany w mię

Fig. 7. E. Korczynski's paper "Coronary artery embolism (*Embolia arteriae coronariae cordis*) diagnosed in a living patient", 1887.

Also the intravital diagnosis of myocardial infarction established by George Dock, an eminent American scientist, being the first such diagnosis recorded in the United States (1896), happened much later than in Europe and nine years after the publication of Korczyński's report.
The immense importance of Professor Korczyński's paper was recognized by a humble Polish internal medicine specialist from Częstochowa, Władysław Biegański, in his textbook (*Differential diagnosis of internal diseases,* 1st edition dated 1891, page 115): "An embolus of one of the major branches of coronary arteries results in an almost instantaneous death. Diagnosing such an embolus intravitally is possible only in certain extremely favorable circumstances. The literature basically reports only two cases of coronary artery occlusion that were diagnosed in a living patient, namely the one described by Hammer and the other - by Korczyński. In the former instance, the occlusion occurred relatively slowly, resulting from a thrombus situated over the semilunar valve and the patient survived for more than 24 hours; in the latter, death occurred within less than 10 minutes, while Professor Korczyński was present in the Department" (Biegański, 1891).

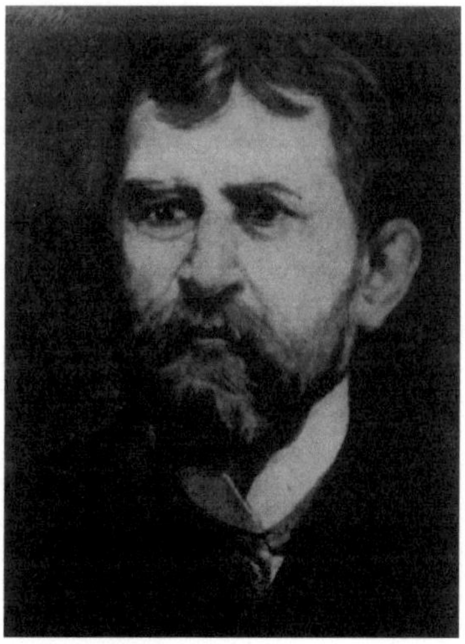

Fig. 8. Władysław Biegański (1857-1917)

Increasingly more often, physicians-practitioners attempted to confirm their diagnoses of angina pectoris by postmortem examinations. They sought lesions involving coronary vessels, more consciously associating necrotic foci of the cardiac muscle with consequences of ischemic heart disease. "Myocardial infarction" was becoming a new diagnosis, not only from the anatomopathological, but also clinical point of view. Pioneering reports in this field also include an early but exquisite paper on myocardial infarction by Józef Pawiński of Warsaw, published in 1883 in the "Gazeta Lekarska" [the Medical Newspaper] and entitled "Coronary artery stenosis and occlusion - a physiological, pathological and clinical view". Pawiński was most assuredly the father of Polish cardiology, its founder on the Polish soil; at the same time, he was a historian of medicine with inclinations towards the humanities; moreover, he deserves the title of a "philosopher of medicine". He was highly valued for his knowledge of pathology and treatment of heart diseases also outside the country (Skalski, 2008).
In 1908, Pawiński wrote in the Pamiętnik Towarzystwa Lekarskiego Warszawskiego [the Memoirs of the Warsaw Medical Society]: "Not only in the history of mankind, but also in

the history of medicine do we find issues that - if we are to understand them precisely - require our going back several centuries. What I mean here is the gradual development of the symptomatology and pathogenesis of *angina pectoris* before Heberden, who in 1768 was the first to present a thorough description of the ailment as a pathological entity and the first to call it *angina pectoris*" (Pawiński, 1908).

Unfortunately, the patients still could not have been offered effective therapy and this was true both for coronary disease and myocardial infarction. Some knowledge was available on the fact that a hygienic lifestyle may prevent episodes of angina pectoris or on how to alleviate pain and thus, even in this modest way, increase the chances of the patient to survive the attack. Thus, opium was employed, along with its derivatives, herbal remedies continued to be recommended due to their anxiolytic, spasmolytic, diuretic and relaxing properties, as well as digitalis and various salts – potassium carbonate, calcium carbonate, magnesium compounds. The turning point in treatment of angina pectoris attacks was the introduction of nitrates. In 1867, a British physician Thomas Lauder Brunton (1844-1916) introduced *Amylium nitrosum*, a medication whose beneficial relaxing properties are unquestionable (Fye, 1986).

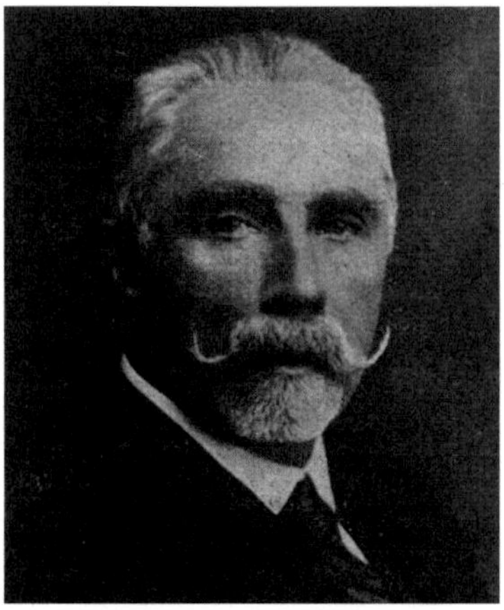

Fig. 9. Józef Pawiński (1851-1925)

Nevertheless, a large-scale employment of nitrates commenced after a British pharmacologist William Murrel (1853-1912) published in 1878/1879 a paper on his experience in using glyceryl trinitrate. Almost immediately after Murrel's report appeared in print, nitroglycerine was introduced in Krakow by E. Korczyński. As soon as only two years later, in 1881, he published his clinical observations of the use of the pharmaceutical. Based on experiments performed jointly with Michał Janocha, Korczyński introduced nitroglycerine to everyday clinical practice, on a large scale at that. He administered 1-6 drops of the drug and observed its effect on the circulatory system that lasted from 3 to 45 minutes, with the most pronounced effect occurring within 3-15 minutes. He described a simultaneous effect exerted on the nervous system and manifested - as reported by the patients - as a sense of warmth appearing inside the head and problems with attention focusing. These are the words Korczyński used while writing about nitroglycerin: " (...) nitroglycerin is a medication which promptly, strongly and almost completely eliminates attacks of stenocardia (...). Most likely, it is also a potent drug that relieves heart palpitations that developed for any reason. If stenocardia or palpitations have no anatomical

grounds, nitroglycerin is capable of completely curing these ailments. In stenocardia with aneurismal background, nitroglycerin is capable of not only temporarily eliminating the attacks, but in rare cases it may to some degree prevent such an attack" (Korczyński, 1881).
In the early 20th century, together with the first experiments with the use of an electrocardiograph developed by Willem Einthoven (1903), the era of increasingly effective clinical diagnostic management began.
In 1912, James Bryan Herrick (1861-1954) of Chicago stated that using the apparatus, one might intravitally establish a firm diagnosis of myocardial infarction and thus autopsy ceased to be the only method of confirming the disease. Indeed, seen from the perspective of the last century, in the history of cardiology, the papers by Herrick should be considered crucial. The possibility of intravital diagnosing myocardial infarction has provided medicine with a chance to modify the available therapy, change general management principles, and finally allowed for determining the prognosis and decrease mortality rates (Herrick, 1912, Acierno & Worrel, 2000).
Subsequent pioneering observations on electrocardiographic diagnosis of myocardial infarction were made by Harold Ensign Bennet Pardee (1886-1973) of New York. In 1920, he presented examples of patients-survivors with a history of myocardial infarction diagnosed based on characteristic ECG recordings (Kligfield, 2005).

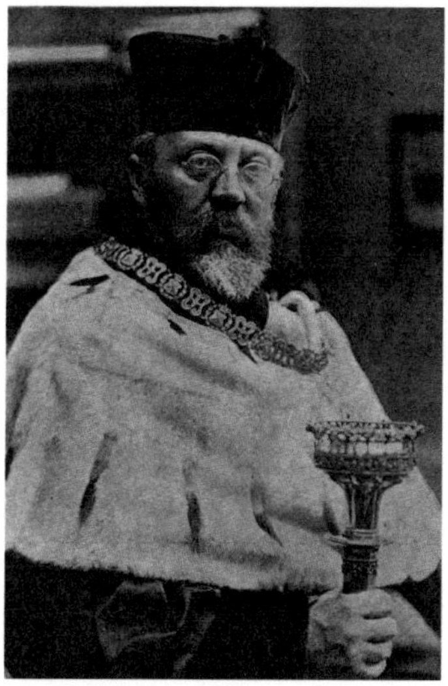

Fig. 10. Napoleon Cybulski (1854-1919)

Poland was not left behind. Soon, the first electrocardiograph was installed in Krakow on the initiative of a Krakow scientist Napoleon Cybulski. Fascinated with the discoveries of Einthoven, Cybulski was the first Polish researcher who obtained in 1910 a recording of electric heart activity, so he is also a pioneer of electrocardiography in Poland (Skalski & Kuch, 2006). He founded a well-known in Europe center of physiological research, and a major part of his studies provided a significant contribution to the development of knowledge on the circulatory system on the international scale. His most important findings, which set foundations for sciences concentrating on arterial hypertension and led to further progress in clinical studies include Cybulski's discovery (jointly with Władysław Szymonowicz) of a substance found in adrenal glands that exhibited potent vasoconstrictive and hypertensive properties (1894). The scientist called the substance in Polish "nadnerczyna" (from the term denoting the adrenal glands) and the name was translated into "adrenalin"(Cybulski, 1895).

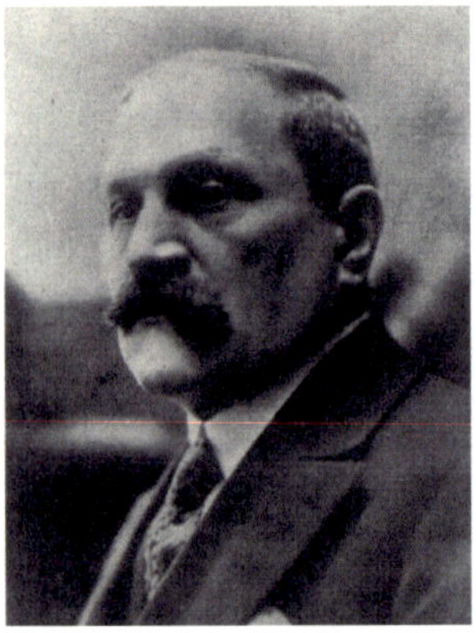

Fig. 11. Józef Latkowski (1873-1948)

In Krakow, also for the first time, Józef Latkowski published a paper that described an ECG recording in pericardial sac obliteration (constrictive pericarditis). The same author presented in 1912 a report that was extraordinary considering it appeared in the initial phase of development of this diagnostic modality, namely "A demonstration of an electrocardiogram from a female patient with *dextrocardia vera*" (Śródka, 2004).

In 1903, Zdzisław Dmochowski published his splendid and extensive textbook entitled "Anatomopathological diagnostics". Obviously, we can find there a modern, reasonable and logical argument focusing on myocardial infarction. Let us quote a fragment: "A gradual growth of intravascular thrombi and their calcification finally lead to pronounced stenosis or a complete occlusion of the vessel. Other condition that causes a complete occlusion of coronary arteries is emboli (*embolia art. coronariae*). This phenomenon is relatively rare and

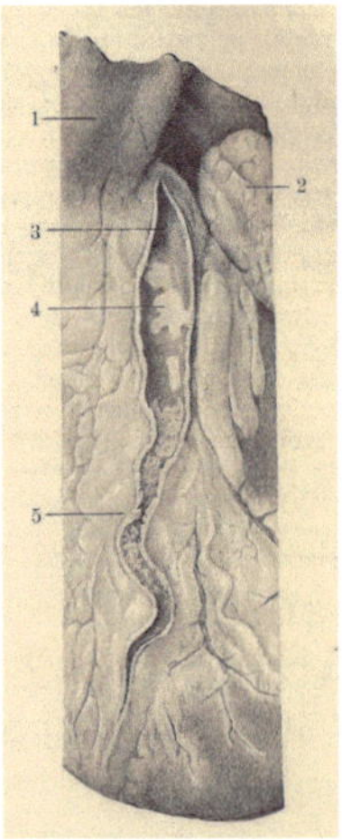

Fig. 12. A presentation of a completely occluded left anterior descending artery from the textbook by Dmochowski (1903).

usually is a complication of acute endocarditis. In such cases, the diagnosis is made based on detecting an embolus. Stenosis or a complete occlusion of coronary arteries strongly affects the cardiac muscle (...). Coronary artery embolus triggers the development of myocardial infarction" (Dmochowski, 1903). In this manner, in the above cited sentence, probably for the first time in the Polish medical literature there appears the term "myocardial infarction". As late as in 1920, the enforced in Europe *International Nomenclature of Diseases and Causes of Death adopted by the International Commission in Paris* (Mianownictwo chorób i przyczyn zgonów..., 1922) did not include "myocardial infarction" at all (it included only an "embolus, thrombus" - without providing information on the location and with the pathologies involving organs other than the heart), not even as the cause of death!

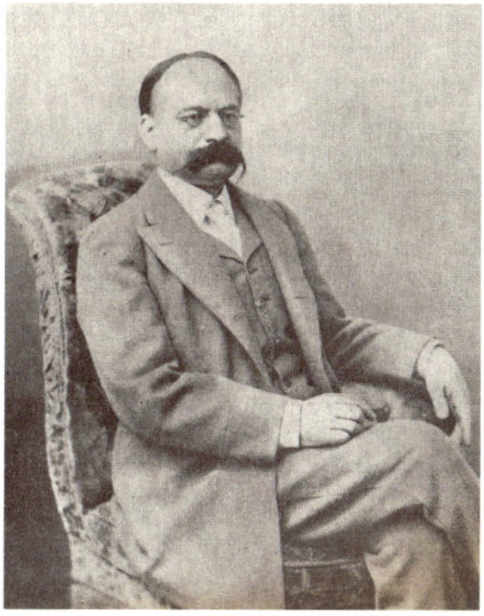

Fig. 13. Walery Jaworski (1849-1924)

In the well-known textbook "The science of internal medicine" edited by Walery Jaworski (Krakow, 1905), a well-executed and extensive chapter on heart diseases written by a student of Korczyński - Antoni Gluziński (1856-1935), a Lvov University, and since 1919 - a Warsaw University professor of internal medicine, also addressed myocardial infarction. Nevertheless, the chapter, 161 pages in length, devoted to myocardial infarction only (or possibly as much as) half a page. Gluziński stated: "Clogging the main coronary artery trunks (...) is the cause of sudden deaths. However, clogging of further situated branches is not as dangerous as it might have been inferred from preliminary experience, and much depends here on the prior status of the cardiac muscle. A consequence of clogging, if there is no sudden death, is the formation of an infarction (*infarctus*), which softens and the heart may rupture at the malacia site (*ruptura cordis*), or else the infarction is absorbed and a larger scar develops at the site (...)"(Gluziński, 1905).
A valuable, although small textbook *Diagnostic management of circulatory organ diseases* authored by a scientist from Lvov Marian Franke presented certain, at that time obligatory knowledge on "angina pectoris" and "cardiac asthma" in condensed, thus entitled chapters. The text is well thought-out, conscientiously written and based on the vast clinical experience of the author. But we also find here a somewhat archaic subject in a chapter "Acute fatigue of the heart" (Franke, 1921). The issue of myocardial infarction is treated by the author as a problem of minor importance only - laconic information on the subject is

squeezed in a small sub-chapter entitled "Embolus and thrombus of the coronary artery", which can be found near the end of the textbook and occupies half a page!
Another important Polish textbook published in the interwar period "Pathology, diagnostics and therapy" (1938), with Feliks Malinowski and Zenon Orłowski as the editors, still provides not enough information on myocardial infarction - at least according to our contemporary expectations. And medicine could then offer insufficiently little help to the patients, although some progress was noticeable. On the issue of treating myocardial infarction (in the chapter authored by Z. Michalski and H. Skwarczewska), the textbook says: "The treatment has three objectives – two immediate (keeping the patient alive and alleviating his pain and general suffering) and subsequently – prevention of new infarctions developing. The first two recommendations require a bed rest with the patient kept as calm as possible for at least 3-4 weeks, i.e. until the necrotic part of the cardiac muscle becomes organized, combined with a simultaneous administration of all types of *excitantia* (camphor and related agents), as well as painkillers. Nitroglycerin is not effective here, most likely it is even noxious, as it decreases blood pressure, which is already low anyway. Large doses of morphine are necessary, although theoretically it is not recommended, since as a vagotonic agent, it causes vessel constriction (...)" (Michalski & Skwarczewska, 1936).

5. Myocardial infarction in the last half of century

In the last decades, the problem of preventing and treating myocardial infarction has become one of major challenges of contemporary medicine. Infarction has long ceased to be a death sentence for the patient; it is merely one of life-threatening conditions that absolutely require immediate medical intervention. The years of Second World War represent stagnation in all sciences, including medicine, both in Poland and in other war-tormented European countries; American medicine might have been affected to a lesser degree, as it was not so much afflicted with the drama of war.
In the post-war years, Polish physicians attempted to keep pace with modern trends in all fields, although in this dark period of our history, successes of our cardiology were seen clearly later in time as compared to Western countries. Nevertheless, in spite of post-war problems and an immense gap in therapeutic possibilities that opened between the Western world and our country, tormented by the war and rampant post-war Communist lawlessness, Polish cardiologists tried to keep pace with progress. In the forties and fifties, successes of Western medicine (predominantly seen in the United States) were carefully followed. As it is apparent - I hope - in the present article, Polish physicians have always been in the forefront of establishing the foundations of world cardiology and this was true both centuries and decades ago. We have to bear in mind what modest diagnostics modalities they had at their disposal - they only had the legacy of pre-war Poland, subject to terrible destruction of the war.
Nevertheless, as early as in 1945, the first Polish reports on problems pertaining to myocardial infarction appeared, authored by Edward Szczeklik. One paper, worthy of particular mention in view of its unique character, concentrated on damages of the heart conduction system in the course of myocardial infarction (Szczeklik, 1945a, 1945b).
Let us emphasize that since the beginning of keeping a register of Polish medical bibliography, doctoral dissertation addressing circulatory system diseases appeared already in the early 19th century (1812). When, then, did the first Polish doctoral theses unquestionably addressing myocardial infarction appear? As it turns out, this happened

only in the post-war period - in 1949 and 1952 (Stanowski, 1949; Jodkowski, 1952; Stawowiak, 1952), and subsequently in 1961 (Smolarz, 1961). However, various problems of circulatory system diseases were relatively frequently the subject of doctoral dissertations (Śródka, 1994).

Physicians found out that the appropriate form of therapeutic management was not exactly the conservative treatment with all pharmacological novelties introduced, fibrinolytic therapy (both intravenous and intracoronary) and adjuvant therapy, but rather restoration of blood flow to the occluded artery. Such a solution of the problem became a milestone in myocardial infarction treatment.

R. G. Favaloro and D. B. Effler were the first to initiate surgical reperfusion in fresh myocardial infarction; in 1971, they published their preliminary observations on this treatment modality (Favaloro et al., 1971). Subsequent reports demonstrated that revascularization in fresh infarction is possible, although associated with a high risk (Cohn et al., 1972; Sanders et al., 1972). In time, the risk related to such a radical and aggressive treatment diminished and in the eighties, the results started to be promising. Mortality rates dropped as low as down to 5%. It became apparent that the major objective of treating fresh myocardial infarction was preservation of cardiac muscle contractility in the infarcted site and - to implement the goal - restoring the patency of the occluded artery.

In Poland, surgical reperfusion in fresh myocardial infarction was introduced by Zbigniew Religa in the Zabrze center in 1985. In 1988 and 1989, Marian Zembala presented his experience in employing this therapeutic modality (Zembala, 1989).

Regardless of progress in surgical treatment of myocardial infarction, in the late seventies, new possibilities emerged of restoring the patency of the occluded artery through a procedure belonging to the realm of modern interventive cardiology. First reports were published describing an attempt at invasive opening of the occlusion from the artery responsible for the zone of infarction (Rentrop et al., 1979) and presenting the first successful results in interventive removal of occlusion of the coronary artery in fresh myocardial infarction (Meyer et al., 1982; Hartzler et al., 1983).

Soon (in 1986), the first in Poland publication on such a therapeutic method authored by M. Dąbrowski et al. appeared in Warsaw (Dąbrowski et al., 1986). At the same time, independently, interventive restoration of patency of the occluded artery in fresh myocardial infarction was introduced in Zabrze.

In the history of medicine, the knowledge on myocardial infarction has been taking shape and maturing as long as there has existed medicine based on intellectual perception of the phenomenon of human health and disease. For centuries and millennia, myocardial infarction was a phenomenon or a quirk of fate that was completely incomprehensible, threatening, even awesome. Later, its mystery was gradually revealed, but still with immense respect and without any genuine confidence that man might change anything in the natural course of the disease.

When we look cross-sectionally on the history of our understanding, diagnosing and treating myocardial infarction, a question arises whether the extraordinary progress of medicine in the 20th and 21st centuries has brought a definitive solution of the problem of treating the condition, whether medicine has finally combated the disease. The answer is "probably not", and the future of myocardial infarction treatment - as is seems today - is associated mostly with genetics and related fields, profound interference with molecular biology within the cell; if revascularization is foreseen in the future, it will have to be completely different that contemporary surgical and interventive procedures. Shall we ever be able to responsibly claim that myocardial infarction, which today we have somehow managed to grasp in the sense of understanding the disease and having therapeutic abilities, is a thing of the past?

6. References

Acierno, L.J. & Worrel, T. (2000). James Bryan Herrick [Profiles in cardiology], *Clin. Cardiol.*, Vol.23, No.4, pp. 230-232, ISSN 0160-9289.

Biegański W. (1891). Diagnostyka Różniczkowa Chorób Wewnętrznych, ed. I, Wydawnictwo Gazety Lekarskiej, Druk K. Kowalewskiego, Warszawa.

Cenner, J. (1820). Dissertatio Inauguralis Medica de Angore Pectoris, Drukarnia M. Dziedzickiego. Kraków.

Chrzczonowicz, J. (1812). Dissertatio inauguralis medica de angore pectoris, Drukarnia Józefa Zawadzkiego. Wilno.

Cohn, L.H.; Gorlin, R.; Herman, M. & Collins, J.J.jr. (1972). Aorto-coronary bypass for acute coronary occlusion, *J. Thorac. Cardiovasc. Surg.* Vol.64, No.4, pp. 503–513, ISSN 0022-5223.

Cybulski, N. (1895). Ueber die Funktion die Nebenniere, Universitäts Buchdruckerei, Krakau.

Dąbrowski, M., Woroszylska, M.; Jodkowski, J.; Chojnowska, L.; Górecka, B.; Sawicki M. & Rużyłło W. (1986). Leczenie ostrego zawału serca przy pomocy przezskórnej śródnaczyniowej koronaroplastyki, *Kardiol. Pol.* Vol.29, No.3, pp. 218-26, ISSN 0022-9032.

Dmochowski, Z. (1903). Dyagnostyka Anatomo-Patologiczna, Wydawnictwo Gazety Lekarskiej, Druk Piotra Laskauera i s-ki, Warszawa.

Domosławski, Z. (1967). Adam Chrystian Thebezjusz. Sławny anatom – fizykiem miejskim w Jeleniej Górze, In: *Rocznik Jeleniogórski*, Vol. 5, pp. 71-76, Wydawnictwo Zakładu Narodowego im. Ossolińskich, Wrocław.

Favaloro, R. G.; Effler, D. B.; Cheanvechai, C.; Quint, R.A. & Sones, F.M. (1971). Acute insufficiency (impeding myocardial infarction and myocardial infarction) surgical treatment by saphenous vein graft technique, *Am. J. Cardiol.*, Vol.28, No.5, pp. 598–607.

Franke, M. (1921). Diagnostyka chorób narządu krążenia, Wydawnictwo Podręczników Uniwersyteckich. Lwów-Warszawa-Kraków.

Fye, W.B. (1986). T. Lauder Brunton and amyl nitrite: a Victorian vasodilator, *Circulation;* Vol.74, No.2, pp. 222-229, ISSN 0009-7322.

Gluziński, A. (1905). Choroby serca i naczyń krwionośnych, In: *Nauka o chorobach wewnętrznych vol. II.* Jaworski W., pp. 278-365, Księgarnia H. Altenberga we Lwowie, Kraków.

Hartzler, G.O.; Rutherford, B.D.; McConahay, D.R.; Johnson, W.L. Jr.; McCallister, B.D.; Gura, G.M.Jr.; Conn, R.C. & Crockett, J.E. (1983). Percutaneous transluminal coronary angioplasty with and without thrombolytic therapy for treatment of acute myocardial infarction, *Am Heart J.*, Vol.106, No. 5, pp: 965-73, ISSN 0002-8703.

Herrick, J.B. (1912). Clinical features of sudden obstruction of the coronary arteries, *JAMA*, 59: 2010-2015.

Janikowski, A. (1844). Skostnienie arteryj koronowych serca. *Pam. Tow. Lek. Warsz.* 11: 78-80.

Jodkowski, H. (1952). O częstości występowania zatorów i zawałów w przebiegu bakteryjnego i przewlekłego zapalenia wsierdzia leczonych penicyliną (doctoral dissertation), Warszawa.

Kligfield, P. (2005). Harold Ensign Bennett Pardee (1886-1973), *Clin. Cardiol.*, Vol.28, No.8, pp. 396-398, ISSN 0160-9289.

Korczyński, E. (1881). Kilka słów o działaniu fizjologicznym i o zastosowaniu leczniczym nitrogliceryny, *Pam. Tow. Lek. Warsz.* 77(4): 609-628.

Korczyński, E. (1887). Zator tętnicy wieńcowej serca (*embolia arteriae coronoriae cordis*) za życia rozpoznany, *Przegl. Lek.*; R26 (1-5): 20-21, 41-43, 57-59, 75-76.

Lie, J.T. (1978). Centenary of the first correct antemortem diagnosis of coronary thrombosis by Adam Hammer (1818–1878): English translation of the original report, *Am. J. Cardiol.* Vol.42, No.5, pp. 849-52, ISSN 0002-9149.

Meyer, J.; Merx, W.; Schmitz, H.; Erbel, R.; Kiesslich, T.; Dorr, R.; Lambertz, H.; Bethege, C.; Krebs, W.; Bardos, P.; Minale, C.; Messmer, B.J. & Effert, S. (1982). Percutaneous transluminal coronary angioplasty immediately after intracoronary streptolysis of transmural myocardial infarction, *Circulation*. Vol.66, No.5, pp. 905-13, ISSN 0009-7322.

Mianownictwo chorób i przyczyn zgonów przyjęte przez Komisję Międzynarodową w Paryżu (1922). Dnia 14.10.1920. Ministerstwo Zdrowia Publicznego, Drukarnia Krajowa W. Krawczyński, E. Egert, Warszawa.

Michalski, Z. & Skwarczewska H. (1936). Zatkanie naczyń wieńcowych. Zawał mięśnia sercowego, In: *Patologia, Diagnostyka i Terapja* Malinowski, F. & Orłowski, Z. Nakładem Warszawskiej Ajencji Wydawniczej "Delta" , Warszawa.

Obrastzow, W.P. & Staschesko, N.D. (1910). Zur Kenntnissder Thrombose der Coronararterien des Herzens, *Ztsch. F. Klin. Med.* 71, 12.

Pamiętnik Jubileuszowy wydany ku uczczeniu dwudziestopięcioletniej działalności Prof. Edwarda Sas Korczyńskiego przez byłych jego uczniów, Drukarnia C.K. Uniwersytetu Jagiellońskiego pod zarządem J. Filipowskiego. Kraków, 1900.

Pawiński, J. (1908). *Angina pectoris* w świetle przeszłości, *Pamiętnik Towarzystwa Lekarskiego Warszawskiego*, Vol.55, pp. 305-307.

Rentrop, K.P.; Blanke, H.; Karsch, K.R. & Kreuzer, H. (1979). Initial experience with transluminal recanalization of the recently occluded infarct-related coronary artery in acute myocardial infarction - comparison with conventionally treated patients. *Clin. Cardiol.* Vol. 2, No.2, pp. 92-105, ISSN 0160-9289.

Richter, Chr. Fr. (1671). Disputatio Inauguralis de Cardialgia (doctoral dissertation), Literis Joannis Nisl., Jena.

Ruciński, Z. & Skalski, J. (2004). Kardiologia w okresie zaborów, In: *Dzieje kardiologii w Polsce na tle kardiologii światowej* Kuch, J. & Śródka, A., pp. 167-227, PWN, ISBN 83-01-14201-4, Warszawa.

Sanders, C.H.A.; Buckley, M.J.; Leinbach, R.C.; Mundth, E.D. & Austen, G.W. (1972). Mechanical circulatory assistance. Current status and experience with combining circulatory assistance emergency coronary angiography and acute myocardial revascularization. *Circulation*. Vol.45, No.7, pp. 1292-1313.

Skalski, J. & Kuch J. (2006). Polish thread in the history of circulatory physiology, *J. Physiol. Pharmacol.*, 57 Supp 1: 5-41.

Skalski, J. & Stembrowicz, W. (2004). Kardiologia w I Rzeczpospolitej In: *Dzieje kardiologii w Polsce na tle kardiologii światowej* Kuch, J. & Śródka, A., pp. 146-166, PWN, ISBN 83-01-14201-4, Warszawa.

Skalski, J. (2009). Niewydolność krążenia w dziejach medycyny, In: *Przewlekła niewydolność serca*, Podolec, P.; Jankowska, E.A.; Ponikowski, P. & Banasiak, W. Medycyna Praktyczna, pp. 30-54, ISBN 978-83-7430-127-5, Kraków.

Skalski, J.; Skalska, A.; Turczyński, B. & Kmieć, K. (2003). Choroba wieńcowa dawniej. Próba oceny wartości pracy *De angore pectoris* Jana Cennera z 1820 roku, w realiach wiedzy współczesnej, *Kardiol. Pol.*, Vol.58, No.4, pp. 282-289, ISSN 0022-9032.

Śliwiński, S. (1976). Tworzenie się podstaw kardiologii w klinice lekarskiej profesora Macieja Brodowicza w Krakowie (1823-1850), *Arch. Hist. Fil. Med.* 39: 41-59.

Smolarz, W. (1961). Analiza wektorów wieńcowych przestrzennych i odprowadzenia dodatkowe jednobiegunowe w EKG w rozpoznaniu przebytych zawałów tylnej ściany serca (doctoral dissertation), Zabrze.

Śródka, A. (1994). Rozprawy doktorskie z zakresu kardiologii na wydziałach lekarskich polskich wyższych uczelni do roku 1974, In: *Dzieje kardiologii w Polsce na tle kardiologii światowej*, Kuch, J. & Śródka, A., pp. 322-331, PWN, ISBN 83-01-11546-7, Warszawa.

Śródka, A. (2004). Kardiologia w okresie międzywojennym, In: *Dzieje kardiologii w Polsce na tle kardiologii światowej* Kuch, J. & Śródka, A., pp. 230-233, PWN, ISBN 83-01-14201-4, Warszawa.

Stanowski, W. J. (1949). Zespół Adams-Stokesa we wczesnym okresie zawału mięśnia sercowego (doctoral dissertation). Kraków.

Stawowiak, S. (1952). Wpływ czynników bioklimatycznych na występowania zawałów serca (doctoral dissertation), Kraków,.

Stembrowicz, W. (1971). Dusznica bolesna w ujęciu historycznym, *Arch. Hist. Fil. Med.* 34: 167-177.

Stembrowicz, W. (1987). Od Heberdena do Pawińskiego i Biegańskiego, *Arch. Hist. Fil. Med.* 50: 33-45.

Stembrowicz, W. (1994). Tomasza z Wrocławia (1297- ok.1378 r.), biskupa tytularnego Sarepty z "Practica Medicinalis XXXIX, De syncopi et debilitate cordis" ("O omdleniu i chorobie serca"), *Arch. Hist. Fil. Med.* 57: 75-82.

Szczeklik, E. (1945a). Przypadek zawału bocznego serca, *Przegl. Lek.*; Vol.1/2, No.6, pp. 129-135.

Szczeklik, E. (1945b). Uszkodzenie układu przewodzącego w zawale sercowym jako objaw umiejscowienia, *Przegl. Lek.*, Vol.1/2, No.9-10, pp. 204-216.

Willius, F.A. & Dry, T.J. (1948). A history of the heart and the circulation, W. B. Saunders Company, Philadelphia.

Zembala, M. (1989). Chirurgiczna reperfuzja mięśnia sercowego w świeżym zawale (a dissertation qualifying the author for assistant professorship), Śląska Akademia Medyczna, Katowice.

Part 2

Diagnostic Techniques

3

Role of Modifier Genes in Idiopathic Cardiomyopathies

Madhu Khullar[1], Bindu Hooda[1] and Ajay Bahl[2]
[1]*Department of Experimental Medicine & Biotechnology*
[2]*Department of Cardiology, Post Graduate Institute of Medical Education and Research,*
Chandigarh
India

But however far we may proceed in analysing the genotypes into separable genes or factors, it must always be borne in mind, that the characters of the organism their phenotypical features are the reaction of the genotype in toto. The Mendelian units as such, taken per se are powerless.
Wilhelm Johannsen, 1923

1. Introduction

Cardiomyopathies are chronic diseases of heart muscle, in which the muscle is abnormally enlarged, thickened, and/or stiffened (1). According to American Heart Association, "*Cardiomyopathies are a heterogeneous group of diseases of the myocardium associated with mechanical and/or electrical dysfunction that usually (but not invariably) exhibit inappropriate ventricular hypertrophy or dilatation and are due to a variety of causes that frequently are genetic. Cardiomyopathies either are confined to the heart or are part of generalized systemic disorders, often leading to cardiovascular death or progressive heart failure related disability*" (1). Within this broad definition, WHO (1995) and International Society & Federation of Cardiology has classified cardiomyopathies into four types:

- Dilated cardiomyopathy (DCM)
- Hypertrophic cardiomyopathy (HCM)
- Restricted cardiomyopathy (RCM)
- Arrhythmogenic right Ventricular cardiomyopathy

2. Dilated cardiomyopathy

Dilated cardiomyopathy (DCM) is the third most common cause of heart failure after coronary artery disease and hypertension with an estimated prevalence of 1:2500 (1, 2). DCM is characterized by a progressive course of ventricular dilatation and systolic dysfunction clinically. The life expectancy is limited and varies according to the underlying etiology. Myocarditis, immunological abnormalities, toxic myocardial damage, and genetic factors are all assumed to be causes. The familial occurrence of DCM, mostly as an autosomal dominant trait, is more common than generally believed. As a matter of fact, 20–30% of all cases of DCM are caused by genetic mutations in sarcomeric and non sarcomeric genes. In the past decade, major progress has been achieved by investigating families with inherited DCM. The analysis of candidate genes led to the discovery of cardiac α-actin, the first DCM-causing gene. In the first report on MYH7 mutations as cause of familial DCM, two different missense mutations were identified in 2 out of 21 families with heritable pure DCM without other organ manifestations. In addition, several groups have described patients who exhibit a conversion from a hypertrophic cardiomyopathy (HCM) to a DCM phenotype. Mutations in TNNT2 seem to lead to complete penetrance and a high proportion of patients die suddenly at younger ages whereas patients with mutations in MYH7 may have a more benign disease course. Mutations in genes encoding sarcomere, cytoskeletal, and nuclear proteins, as well as proteins involved in regulation of Ca^{2+} metabolism have been found to be associated with DCM (6-16). When considering the contribution of all known DCM genes, it is estimated that mutations in known disease genes are the cause of inherited DCM in approximately 20% of cases. This low proportion reflects a more complicated genetic etiology than assumed.

3. Hypertrophic cardiomyopathy

HCM is a mendelian trait with an autosomal dominant pattern of familial inheritance whose clinical diagnosis is based on the identification of increased wall thickness of left ventricle in absence of loading conditions (hypertension and valve disease) (17, 18). Mostly based on studies performed until the late 1980s, HCM was originally described and perceived as a rare disease. Later subsequent studies revealed HCM as an epidemiologically relevant, widespread, yet infrequently diagnosed condition. These studies, however, were run according to different designs: some utilized echocardiography as a screening tool of large populations and should thus be considered as true prevalence studies, while others reported data from large group of subjects referred to echocardiography according to different criteria and protocols. Thus, this latter group of studies may have underestimated the prevalence of HCM as small fraction of the originally screened individuals was subsequently referred to echocardiography. From these studies HCM emerges as an important global disease affecting approximately 1:500 individuals worldwide, and is the most common cause of sudden death in the young (3).

The disease seems to be sporadic in ~ 50% of cases but the incomplete penetrance of the phenotype in carriers of some mutations could lead to underestimation of the percentage of familial cases. It is now known that HCM is genetically heterogeneous and caused by mutation in any one of the genes that encode contractile proteins of the cardiac sarcomere, involving thick filaments and thin filaments and in cardiac myosin binding protein C - the structural network that joins thick and thin filaments (17, 19-22). Hundreds of mutations in more than a dozen genes that encode protein constituents of the sarcomere have been identified in HCM (23, 24). MYH7, MYBPC3, TNNI3 and cardiac troponin T (TNNT2) are the most prevalent disease genes, but mutations have also been found in α-tropomyosin (TPM1), cardiac actin (ACTC), cardiac troponin C (TNNC1), essential myosin light chain (MYL3), regulatory myosin light chain (MYL2), α-cardiac myosin heavy chain (MYH6), titin (TTN), γ2 subunit of the protein kinase A (PRKAG2). The prognosis of HCM varies considerably with respect to the reported mutations.

4. Restrictive cardiomyopathy

Restrictive cardiomyopathy (RCM) is an uncommon myocardial disease characterized by increased stiffness of ventricles leading to impaired filling of blood in the presence of normal wall thickness and systolic function. Most affected individuals have severe signs and symptoms of heart failure. RCM may present with interventricular conduction delays, heart block, or skeletal muscle disease. However, the diagnostic criteria for restriction are not universally accepted, and the morphology generally overlaps with HCM, often making the diagnosis difficult.

Previously, RCM was believed to be of idiopathic origin unless otherwise associated with inflammatory, infiltrative or systemic disease but now the results of recent molecular genetic investigations have revealed that a substantial proportion of RCM (not associated with systemic disease) is caused by mutations in sarcomeric disease genes that have been associated with HCM and DCM (25-29).

5. Arrhythmogenic right ventricular cardiomyopathy

Arrhythmogenic Right Ventricular cardiomyopathy/Dysplasia (ARVD) is a cardiomyopathy characterized by progressive degeneration and fibrous-fatty replacement of right ventricular myocardium, by arrhythmias with a left branch block pattern and by increased risk of sudden death in juveniles. The prevalence of ARVD has been estimated to be 1 in 5,000. Several forms of dominant arrhythmogenic right ventricular cardiomyopathy/dysplasia have been identified so far: ARVD1 (14q24.3), ARVD2 (1q42), ARVD3 (14q11-q12), ARVD4 (2q32), ARVD5 (3p23), ARVD6 (10p12-p14) and ARVD7 (10q22). Mutations in the genes encoding the cardiac ryanodine receptor were detected in patients affected with ARVD2.11 (30, 31). Attempts to identify genes involved in other dominant ARVDs were so far unsuccessful.

6. Modifier genes

In many genetic disorders in which a primary disease-causing locus has been identified, evidence exists for additional trait variation due to genetic factors. These findings have led to studies seeking secondary 'modifier' loci. Identification of modifier loci provides insight into disease mechanisms and may provide additional screening and treatment targets. Genetic background, often referred to as the modifier genes, do not cause the disease but simply affects the severity of its phenotypic expression particularly in case of autosomal dominant disorders in which age-dependent onset and variable expressivity are characteristic. The final phenotype is the result of interactions between the causal genes, genetic background (modifier genes), and probably the environmental factors.

One of the major features of cardiomyopathies is a wide phenotypic heterogeneity among affected subjects, which is characterized by variable degree or distribution of hypertrophy and prognosis in HCM patients and variable penetrance of disease in DCM patients carrying same mutations. Part of this can be explained by locus heterogeneity but genetic studies have revealed the presence of clinically healthy individuals carrying the mutant allele, which is, in first-degree relatives, associated with a typical phenotype of the disease. This variable expressivity suggests the existence of modifier genes or polymorphisms, which modulate the phenotypic expression of the disease. Obvious candidate modifier genes encode proteins implicated in cardiac growth and hypertrophy. Several components of the renin–angiotensin–aldosterone system (RAAS) and adrenergic signaling pathways have been analyzed in patients with idiopathic cardiomyopathies. In fact genetic variations in these genes might be one explanation for the well known inter-individual variations in drug responses (ACE inhibitors and beta blockers) in patients.

In this chapter, we have provided information on association of several candiadate genes with clinical phenotype of cardiomyopathies. We identified studies of modifier genes from PubMed search using the MESH terms 'cardiomyopathy and genetics or genetic polymorphisms, or MESH terms Modifier genes and cardiomyopathy or heart failure, limiting results to the English language publications on studies in human adults. We further identified specific polymorphisms of interest noted in earlier reviews and performed additional PubMed searches based on these candidate genes. Our aim was to collate the existing body of knowledge on common genetic polymorphisms and their relationship to phenotypic expression of cardiomyopathy. We have included information on individual study size and design, as well as the strength of statistical association. We tried to remove bias in the selection of research articles by selecting maximum number of studies and from different ethnic groups and by reviewing both published and unpublished (where ever possible) data. The reference lists of all articles obtained were examined to identify additional studies. All titles and abstracts from the search process were examined. The retrieved studies were examined and included if: 1) the patients were well characterized for cardiomyopathies i.e. LVEF ≤40% for DCM and LVH (septal thickness) >13mm for HCM and 2) Results were compared with well categorized control samples.

7. Renin Angiotensin System genes as modifiers in idiopathic cardiomyopathies

The classical renin-angiotensin system (RAS) consists of renin, angiotensin-converting enzyme, angiotensinogen and its receptors. Renin is synthesized in the kidney, stored in the afferent arterioles and released in response to hemodynamic, neurogenic, and ionic signals. Renin, has a very high specificity for its substrate angiotensinogen (AGT). Renin cleaves AGT to release the amino terminal decapeptide angiotensin I (Ang I). Angiotensin-converting enzyme (ACE), which is expressed endothelially, then cleaves Ang I to release the two carboxy terminal amino acids. The resulting octapeptide is designated angiotensin II (Ang II). Ang I is biologically inactive while Ang II is a potent vasoconstrictor. The members of RAS pathway acting as modifier genes will be described in this chapter.

8. Angiotensin Converting Enzyme (ACE)

Angiotensin I-converting enzyme (ACE), is a dipeptidyl peptidase transmembrane-bound enzyme (32). A soluble form of ACE in plasma is derived from the plasma membrane-bound form by proteolytic cleavage of its COOH-terminal domain. There are two distinct isoforms of ACE: somatic and testicular. They are transcribed from a single gene at different initiation sites. The somatic form of ACE is a large protein (150–180 kDa) that has two identical catalytic domains and a cytoplasmic tail. It is synthesized by the vascular endothelium and by several epithelial and neural cell types. The testicular form of ACE is a 100- to 110-kDa protein that has a single catalytic domain corresponding to the COOH-terminal domain of somatic ACE and is only found in developing spermatids and mature sperm where it may play a role in fertilization. It has two primary functions:

- ACE catalyses the conversion of AngI to AngII, a potent vasoconstrictor
- ACE degrades bradykinin, a potent vasodilator, and other vasoactive peptides, (33)

These two actions make ACE inhibition a goal in the treatment of conditions such as high blood pressure, heart failure, diabetic nephropathy, and type 2 diabetes mellitus. Inhibition of ACE (by ACE inhibitors) results in the decreased formation of AngII and decreased metabolism of bradykinin, leading to systematic dilation of the arteries and veins and a decrease in arterial blood pressure. In addition, inhibiting AngII formation diminishes AngII-mediated aldosterone secretion from the adrenal cortex, leading to a decrease in water and sodium reabsorption and a reduction in extracellular volume (34).

Genetic variations in ACE gene have been reported to be associated with many cardiovascular diseases including cardiomyopathies. An insertion or deletion of a 287bp DNA fragment in the ACE gene (ACEI/D) has been found to be an important modifier which may influence the clinical phenotype in cardiomyopathies. ACE I/D polymorphism has been shown to be associated with left ventricular hypertrophy (LVH) in untreated hypertension, complications of atherosclerosis (35) and HCM (36- 40). D allele was shown to be associated with increased risk of cardiomyopathy in Asian Indians; HCM patients with DD genotype were found to be more susceptible to disease (38). D allele carrying genotypes (DD, ID) were also found to be associated with higher mean septal thickness as compared to II genotype in HCM patients, however, the difference was not significant (P>0.05). DCM patients with ID genotype also showed significantly decreased left ventricular ejection fraction (LVEF) indicating a possible association of D allele in pathogenesis of DCM. It has been suggested that DD genotype may be an important biomarker of HCM and presence of the ACE gene I/D polymorphism may be an important marker to identify those individuals with HCM who are likely to have more progressive disease, and therefore at higher risk of adverse clinical outcomes (38, 39). DD-ACE is considered a 'pro-LVH' modifier in HCM (41). DD genotype has been shown to be associated with increased tissue levels of ACE resulting in increased AngII which may lead to increased hypertrophy and fibrosis.

9. Angiotensinogen (AGT)

AGT is an inactive peptide of Renin-Angiotensin System that is produced constitutively and released into the circulation mainly by the liver. Gene for AGT is located on chromosome 1 and codes for 452 amino acids. The first 12 amino acids are the most important for activity. Angiotensinogen is converted into bioactive Angiotensin II, mainly by the action of Renin and ACE.

Given the importance of AGT as a substrate for generation for vasoconstrictive AngII, it has been used as a therapeutic target in heart failure (HF). Genetic variations of this gene have been suggested to represent a predisposing factor to heart failure. Two single nucleotide polymorphisms (SNPs) in AGT (T174M and M235T) have been shown to be associated with HF; for example, an increased frequency of the AGT T235 allele and the AGT 235TT genotype has been reported in HCM associated HF. Rigat et al (1990) have studied AGT polymorphism in 111 healthy volunteers and 58 HF patients with a documented left ventricular ejection fraction (LVEF) ≤40% within the previous 6 months. And observed mutant T allele (T235) to be more prevalent in HF group as compared to healthy controls (*P* = 0.0025, OR 2.02, 95% CI 1.24, 3.30); AGT haplotype (174M and 235T) was also found to be associated with the HF phenotype (*P* = 0.0069) (45). An evaluation of gene-gene interactions revealed significant interaction between AGT (T235) and ACED polymorphisms in the HF group (*P* = 0.02, OR 2.12, 95% CI 1.11, 4.06) suggesting that AGT/ACE gene combination may play an important role in disease predisposition (43). Since polymorphisms of the ACE gene can modulate the circulating AngII levels (42), thus co occurrence of risk alleles of both ACE and AGT genes could be associated with left ventricular hypertrophy (LVH).

AngII, along with pressure overload, has been shown to play a key role in myocardial fibrosis (one of the key features in HCM) by regulation of synthesis of fibrillar collagen in cardiac fibroblasts (44). However, several studies failed to find an association between AGT M235T polymorphism and risk of heart failure (45, 46). Thus, role of these genetic polymorphisms as determinants of disease phenotype (i.e. LVH) still remains to be confirmed.

10. Angiotensin Receptors (AGTR)

AGTRs are a class of G protein-coupled receptors . There are two types of angiotensin receptors: Angiotensin Receptor Type1 (AGTR1) and Angiotensin Receptor Type2 (AGTR2). AGTR1 and AGTR2 receptors share a sequence identity of ~30%, but have a similar affinity for AngII, which is their main ligand.
The AGTR1 receptor belongs to the G protein-coupled receptor (GPCR) superfamily and is primarily coupled through G proteins to the activation of phospholipase C and calcium signaling. The AGTR1 receptors mediate virtually all of the known physiological actions of AngII in cardiovascular, renal, neuronal, endocrine, hepatic, and other target cells. These actions include the regulation of arterial blood pressure, electrolyte and water balance, thirst, hormone secretion, and renal function. The gene coding for AGTR1 is located on chromosome 3 and codes for 359 amino acids. A single nucleotide polymorphism A1166C in 3′ UTR of AGTR1 gene has been found to be associated with increased left ventricular mass without hypertension (47). Arthur et al showed that the AGTR1 genotype influenced the magnitude of LVH in subjects with HCM and it was significantly higher in patients carrying risk 'C' allele genotypes than in AA homozygotes, so proposed that A/C1166 polymorphism could modulate the phenotypic expression of hypertrophy in subjects with HCM and may explain why individuals with the same HCM mutation show a significant variability in the magnitude of LVH (48).

11. Adrenergic receptor genes as modifiers in idiopathic cardiomyopathies

Adrenergic receptors mediate the central and peripheral actions of the neurohormones epinephrine and norepinephrine. Stimulation of adrenergic receptors by catecholamines released from sympathetic branch of autonomic nervous system results in a variety of effects such as increased heart rate, regulation of vascular tone and bronchodilation. In the central nervous system, adrenergic receptors are involved in many functions including memory, learning, alertness and the response to stress.
β-Adrenoceptors (β-AR) are expressed in many cell types throughout the body and play a pivotal role in regulation of cardiac, pulmonary, vascular, endocrine and central nervous system. Although originally adrenergic receptors were divided into two types: α and β, but later on depending on the pharmacological differences these were further divided into many subtypes.
Several different subtypes of β-ARs have been reported in the myocardium and many functionally relevant polymorphisms in the genes encoding for these receptor subtypes have been identified (49). The β1-AR is the dominant subtype and represents 70-80% of β-ARs in the non failing heart (50); β2-AR represents 20-40% (51). In vascular smooth muscle the majority of β-ARs are β2AR. Desensitization and downregulation of adrenergic receptors are principal mechanism observed in heart failure. Desensitization is the mechanism by which cells decrease effector responses, despite the presence of ligands; this is usually due to

defect in G-protein coupling. In heart failure, both β1-AR and β2-AR are significantly desensitized due to uncoupling of receptor from its respective signaling pathways (52, 53). Several SNPs in both β1-AR (ADRB1) and β2-AR (ADRB2) genes have been examined for association with HF. Two (ADRB1) SNPs Ser49Gly and Arg389Gly have been commonly studied for association with HF (54). Cinzia et al. showed that the β1-AR Gly49 variant and the β2-AR Gly16Gly genotypes were significantly and independently associated with the DCM phenotype (55). We have examined association of ADRB2 Gln27Glu polymorphism in modulating the phenotypic variability in patients diagnosed with idiopathic cardiomyopathies in Asian Indian patients and observed that HCM patients with mutant Glu27 allele had lower mean septal thickness as compared to carriers of wild type allele but the results lacked statistical significance (p>0.05). DCM patients with 27Glu allele also showed decreased LVEF indicating a possible role of this polymorphism in pathogenesis of DCM. Another polymorphism (ADRB2 Q27E), however, was not found to be associated or influence phenotypic variability of the idiopathic cardiomyopathies in the same cohort (unpublished data). In vitro studies have indicated that these SNPs result in variation in the receptor coupling to stimulatory G (Gs)-protein or agonist-promoted receptor downregulation (56-60). Unlike the β1-AR, the β2-AR does not undergo down regulation in failing myocardium, but may account for about 40% of surface receptors (61). It has been proposed that changes in the expression or properties of the β-adrenergic receptors due to single nucleotide polymorphism (SNPs) might influence cardiovascular function or may contribute to the pathophysiology of several disorders like hypertension, congestive heart failure, asthma, obesity or type 2 diabetes mellitus.

12. Other modifier genes in cardiomyopathies

Recently several other genes such as ACE2, Calmodulin III and TnnI3K have been also studied for their role as modifier genes in cardiomyopathies.

13. Angiotensin Converting Enzyme 2 (ACE2)

Angiotensin-converting enzyme 2 (ACE2) is a homolog of ACE, and hydrolyzes Ang I to produce Ag-(1-9), which is subsequently converted into Ang-(1-7) by a neutral endopeptidase and ACE. ACE2 releases Ang-(1-7) more efficiently than its catalysis of Ang-(1-9). Thus, the major biologically active product of ACE2 is Ang-(1-7), which is considered to be a beneficial peptide of the RAS cascade in the cardiovascular system (62, 63). ACE2 is present in a wide variety of cells including heart (64-68). ACE2 is a carboxy-monopeptidase with a preference for hydrolysis between a proline and carboxy-terminal hydrophobic or basic residues, differing from ACE, which cleaves two amino acids from AngI. ACE inhibitors have no direct effect on ACE2 activity. As a result, ACE2 is a central enzyme in balancing vasoconstrictor and proliferative actions of AngII with vasodilatory and antiproliferative effects of Ang-(1-7) (66, 69).
Genetic variants in the ACE2 have been recently shown to be associated with left ventricular mass, and LVH in hemizygous men (70). Two mutant alleles of ACE2 SNPs (rs2106809 and rs6632677) have been also found to be associated with increased risk of HCM. An ACE2 haplotype comprising of mutant alleles of these two SNPs was found to be associated with 1.59 fold increased risk of HCM in male patients (71). These observations suggest that ACE2 genotypes may be important determinants of quantum of LVH in patients with HCM.

14. Calmodulin gene

Proteins involved in hypertrophic pathways or mediators of Ca2+ signaling in cardiomyocytes are promising candidates as modifier genes (72, 73). Calmodulin (CaM) is a ubiquitous, highly conserved Ca^{2+} sensor involved in the regulation of a wide variety of cellular events. Many of the actions of Ca2+ are mediated through its interaction with calmodulin (CaM), which serves as an intracellular sensor for Ca2+ ions and plays a major role in Ca2+ homeostasis. Thus, any genetic variant that directly affect CaM gene expression and/or function would be expected to impact on the intracellular Ca2+ concentration. In humans, CaM is encoded by a multigene family consisting of three members, CALM1, CALM2, and CALM3, which are located on chromosomes 14q24–q31, 2p21.1–p21.3, and 19q13.2–q13.3.22. A -34 T>A polymorphism in the 5′-flanking region of human CALM3 gene has been shown to be differently distributed between familial HCM (FHC) patients and controls and between affected and healthy carriers of an FHC mutation indicating that -34 T>A CALM3 polymorphism is a potential modifier gene for FHC in patients carrying a mutation in either the MYH7 or MYBPC3 gene (74).

15. Cardiac Troponin I-interacting kinase

Cardiac troponin I-interacting kinase (Tnni3k) is a novel cardiac specific protein kinase that interacts with cardiac Troponin I (cTnI) (75). A yeast two hybrid interaction screen with a C-terminal fragment of Tnni3k identified several additional sarcomeric proteins as putative binding partners such as cardiac α-actin and myosin binding protein C (76). Wheeler et al showed that a 3784(C>T) polymorphism in intron 19 in Tnni3k coding gene activates a cryptic splice site, generating an aberrant transcript that undergoes NMD (Nonsense Mediated Decay), leading to drastically reduced mRNA levels and an apparent absence of Tnni3k protein. Their study showed that Tnni3k might modulate sarcomere function through interactions with key components of the sarcomeric complex (77). However, the role of TNNI3K polymorphisms in modulating phenotype of cardiomyopathy patients is not well studied and needs to be examined in different ethnic populations.

16. Modifier genes as potential therapeutic interventions in cardiomyopathies

Cardiomyopathies are emerging as a frequent cause of hospitalization and mortality among men and women world wide. Traditional risk factors and mutations in causal genes alone cannot fully account for the inter-individual variation in the prevalence and penetrance of the disease in general population. Identification of modifier loci provides insight into disease mechanisms and may provide additional screening and treatment targets.

Recent studies suggest that pharmacologic blockade of modifier genes could confer beneficial effects in cardiomyopathies, such as relief in symptoms (syncope, dyspnea, LVEF etc.). ACE inhibitors, Angiotensin Receptor Blockers (ARBs) and beta blockers are now part of routine therapy for hypertension, heart failure and myocardial infarction (MI). They reduce the risk of all cardiovascular events and all-cause mortality by reducing blood pressure makes it easier for the heart to pump blood and can improve heart failure.

Apart from the pharmacological modulations of modifier genes, many trials on gene therapy and animal models of the disease are on going which will provide better understanding of the pathophysiology of cardiomyopathies and will also help in better patient management. For example, pharmacologic interventions in transgenic animal

models of HCM aimed at the potential modifier genes have highlighted the role of modifier genes in the pathogenesis of morphologic and histological phenotypes in HCM. Lim et al showed that blockade of AGTR1 in the cardiac troponin T-Q92 transgenic mouse model reduced interstitial collagen volume by 49% and expression of collagen (I) mRNA and transforming growth factor, a known mediator of profibrotic effects of angiotensin II, by approximately 50% (78). Because interstitial fibrosis is considered a major risk factor for SCD and ventricular arrhythmias in human patients with HCM (69, 79), it illustrates that interventions aimed at the modifier genes could reduce the severity of the phenotype (myocardial fibrosis, LVH, risk of SCD) and mortality in idiopathic cardiomyopathies.
To conclude, along with identification of mutations in causal genes, delineation of genetic variations in modifier genes is needed to understand the pathogenesis of the cardiomyopathies and for symptomatic treatment of the patients. This approach will be helpful for personalized medicine as etiology and severity of idiopathic cardiomyopathies is highly variable in patients.

17. References

[1] Maron BJ, Towbin JA, Thiene G, Antzelevitch C, Corrado D, Arnett D et al. Contemporary definitions and classification of the cardiomyopathies: an American Heart Association Scientific Statement from the Council on Clinical Cardiology, Heart Failure and Transplantation Committee; Quality of Care and Outcomes Research and Functional Genomics and Translational Biology Interdisciplinary Working Groups; and Council on Epidemiology and Prevention. Circulation 2006;113(14):1807-16.
[2] Abelmann WH. Classification and natural history of primary myocardia Disease. Prog Cardiovasc Dis 1984;27(2):73-94.
[3] Maron BJ, Shirani J, Poliac LC, Mathenge R, Roberts WC, Mueller FO. Sudden death in young competitive athletes: Clinical, demographic, and pathological profiles. Jama 1996;276(3):199-204.
[4] Olson TM, Michels VV, Thibodeau SN, Tai YS, Keating MT. Actin mutations in dilated cardiomyopathy, a heritable form of heart failure. Science 1998;280:750–752.
[5] Kamisago M, Sharma SD, DePalma SR, Solomon S, Sharma P, McDonough B, Smoot L, Mullen MP, Woolf PK, Wigle ED, Seidman JG, Seidman CE, Jarcho J, Shapiro LR. Mutations in sarcomere protein genes as a cause of dilated cardiomyopathy. N Engl J Med 2000; 343:1688–1696.
[6] Arbustini E, Pilotto A, Repetto A, Grasso M, Negri A, Diegoli M et al. Autosomal dominant dilated cardiomyopathy with atrioventricular block: a lamin A/C defect-related disease. J Am Coll Cardiol 2002;39(6):981-90.
[7] Murphy RT, Mogensen J, Shaw A, Kubo T, Hughes S, McKenna WJ. Novel mutation in cardiac troponin I in recessive idiopathic dilated Cardiomyopathy. Lancet 2004;363(9406):371-2.
[8] Daehmlow S, Erdmann J, Knueppel T, Gille C, Froemmel C, Hummel M et al. Novel mutations in sarcomeric protein genes in dilated cardiomyopathy. Biochem Biophys Res Commun 2002;298(1):116-20.
[9] Hanson EL, Jakobs PM, Keegan H, Coates K, Bousman S, NH Dienel, Litt M, Hershberger RE. Cardiac troponin T lysine 210 deletion in a family with dilated cardiomyopathy. J Card Fail 2002;8(1):28-32.

[10] Knoll R, Hoshijima M, Hoffman HM, Person V, Lorenzen-Schmidt I, Bang ML et al. The cardiac mechanical stretch sensor machinery involves a Z disc complex that is defective in a subset of human dilated cardiomyopathy. Cell 2002;111(7):943-55.

[11] Olson TM, Illenberger S, Kishimoto NY, Huttelmaier S, Keating MT, Jockusch BM. Metavinculin mutations alter actin interaction in dilated Cardiomyopathy. Circulation 2002;105(4):431-7.

[12] Schmitt JP, Kamisago M, Asahi M, Li GH, Ahmad F, Mende U et al. Dilated cardiomyopathy and heart failure caused by a mutation in phospholamban. Science 2003;299(5611):1410-13.

[13] McNair WP, Ku L, Taylor MR, Fain PR, Dao D, Wolfel E, Mestroni L. SCN5A mutation associated with dilated cardiomyopathy, conduction disorder, and arrhythmia. Circulation 2004;110(15):2163-7.

[14] Bienengraeber M, Olson TM, Selivanov VA, Kathmann EC, O'Cochlain F, F Gao et al. ABCC9 mutations identified in human dilated cardiomyopathy disrupt catalytic KATP channel gating. Nat Genet 2004;36(4):382-7.

[15] Tsubata S, Bowles KR, Vatta M, Zintz C, Titus J, Muhonen L et al. Mutations in the human delta-sarcoglycan gene in familial and sporadic dilated cardiomyopathy. J Clin Invest 2000;106(5):655-62.

[16] Olson TM, Michels VV, Thibodeau SN, Tai YS, Keating MT. Actin mutations in dilated cardiomyopathy, a heritable form of heart failure. Science 1998;280(5364):750-2.

[17] Marian AJ, Roberts R. Recent advances in the molecular genetics of hypertrophic cardiomyopathy. Circulation 1995;92(5):1336-47.

[18] Schwartz K, Carrier L, Guicheney P, Komajda M. Molecular basis of familial cardiomyopathies. Circulation 1995;91(2):532-40.

[19] Ciro E, Nichols PF, Maron BJ. Heterogeneous morphologic expression of genetically transmitted hypertrophic cardiomyopathy. Two dimensional echocardiographic analysis. Circulation 1983;67(6):1227-33.

[20] Coviello DA, Maron BJ, Spirito P, Watkins H, Vosberg HP, Thierfelder L et al. Clinical features of hypertrophic cardiomyopathy caused by mutation of a "hot spot" in the alpha-tropomyosin gene. J Am Coll Cardiol 1997;29(3):635-40.

[21] Watkins H, Rosenzweig A, Hwang DS, Levi T, McKenna W, Seidman CE, Seidman JG. Characteristics and prognostic implications of myosin missense mutations in familial hypertrophic cardiomyopathy. N Engl J Med 1992;326(17):1108-14.

[22] Niimura H, Bachinski LL, Sangwatanaroj S, Watkins H, Chudley AE, McKenna W et al. Mutations in the gene for cardiac myosin-binding protein C and late-onset familial hypertrophic cardiomyopathy. N Engl J Med 1998;338(18):1248-57.

[23] Richard P, Charron P, Carrier L, Ledeuil C, Cheav T, Pichereau C et al. Hypertrophic cardiomyopathy: distribution of disease genes, spectrum of mutations, and implications for a molecular diagnosis strategy. Circulation 2003;107(17):2227-32.

[24] Rai TS, Ahmad S, Bahl A, Ahuja M, Ahluwalia TS, Singh B et al. Genotype phenotype correlations of cardiac beta-myosin heavy chain mutations in Indian patients with hypertrophic and dilated cardiomyopathy. Mol Cell Biochem 2009;321:189–96.

[25] Rai TS, Ahmad S, Ahluwalia TS, Ahuja M, Bahl A, Saikia UN et al. Genetic and clinical profile of Indian patients of idiopathic restrictive cardiomyopathy with and without hypertrophy. Mol Cell Biochem. 2009;331(1-2):187-92.

[26] Hughes SE, McKenna WJ. New insights into the pathology of inherited Cardiomyopathy. Heart 2005;91(2):257-64.
[27] Zhang J, Kumar A, Stalker HJ, Virdi G, Ferrans VJ, Horiba K et al. Clinical and molecular studies of a large family with desmin-associated restrictive cardiomyopathy. Clin Genet 2001;59(4):248-56.
[28] Mogensen J, Kubo T, Duque M, Uribe W, Shaw A, Murphy R et al. Idiopathic restrictive cardiomyopathy is part of the clinical expression of cardiac troponin I mutations. J Clin Invest 2003;111(2):209-16.
[29] Peddy SB, Vricella LA, Crosson JE, Oswald GL, Cohn RD et al. Infantile restrictive cardiomyopathy resulting from a mutation in the cardiac troponin T gene. Pediatrics 2006;117(5):1830-33.
[30] Hendrik Milting H, Lukas N, Klauke B, Körfer R, Perrot A, Osterziel KJ et al. Composite polymorphisms in the ryanodine receptor 2 gene associated with arrhythmogenic right ventricular cardiomyopathy. Cardiovasc Res 2006;71(3):496-505.
[31] Bauce B, Rampazzo A, Basso C, Bagattin A, Daliento L, Tiso N et al. Screening for ryanodine receptor type 2 mutations in families with effort-induced polymorphic ventricular arrhythmias and sudden death: Early diagnosis of asymptomatic carriers. J Am Coll Cardiol 2002;40(2):341-349.
[32] Walter F, The Adrenal Gland. *Medical Physiology: A Cellular And Molecular Approaoch* 2003;1059.
[33] Imig JD. ACE Inhibition and Bradykinin-Mediated Renal Vascular Responses: EDHF Involvement. *Hypertension* 2004;43(3):533–5.
[34] Klabunde RE. ACE-inhibitors. *Cardiovasc Pharmacol Concepts* 2009. cvpharmacology.com. http://www.cvpharmacology.com/vasodilator/ACE.htm.
[35] Wang JG, Staessen JA. Genetic polymorphisms in the renin–angiotensin system: relevance for susceptibility to cardiovascular disease. Eur J Pharm 2000;410:289–302.
[36] Lechin M, Quinones MA, Omran A, Hill R, Yu QT, Rakowski H et al. Angiotensin-I converting enzyme genotypes and left ventricular hypertrophy in patients with hypertrophic cardiomyopathy. Circulation 1995;92:1808–12.
[37] Ortlepp JR, Vosberg HP, Reith S, Ohme F, Mahon NG, Schroder D et al. Genetic polymorphisms in the renin–angiotensin–aldosterone system associated with expression of left ventricular hypertrophy in hypertrophic cardiomyopathy: a study of five polymorphic genes in a family with a disease causing mutation in the myosin binding protein C gene. Heart 2002;87:270–75.
[38] Rai TS, Dhandapany PS, Ahluwalia TS, Bhardwaj M, Bahl A, Talwar KK, Khullar M et al. ACE I/D polymorphism in Indian patients with hypertrophic cardiomyopathy and dilated cardiomyopathy. Mol Cell Biochem 2008;311:67–72.
[39] Doolan G, Nguyen L, Chung J, Ingles J, Semsarian C. Progression of left ventricular hypertrophy and the angiotensinconverting enzyme gene polymorphism in hypertrophic cardiomyopathy. Int J Cardiol 2004;96(2):157–163.
[40] Schut AF, Bleumink GS, Stricker BH, Hofman A, Witteman JC, Pols HA, Deckers JW et al. Angiotensin converting enzyme insertion/deletion polymorphism and the risk of heart failure in hypertensive subjects. Eur Heart J 2004;25(23):2143–8.

[41] Tesson F, Dufour C, Moolman JC, Carrier L, al-Mahdawi S, Chojnowska L et al. The influence of the angiotensin I converting enzyme genotype in familial hypertrophic cardiomyopathy varies with the disease gene mutation. J Mol Cell Cardiol 1997;29:831–8.

[42] Rigat B, Hybert C, Alhenc-Gelas F. An insertion/ deletion polymorphism of angiotensin I converting enzyme accounting for half of the variance of the serum enzyme levels. J Clin Invest 1990; 86: 1343–6.

[43] Zakrzewski JM, de Denus S, Dubé MP, François B, White M, Turgeon J. Ten renin-angiotensin system-related gene polymorphisms in maximally treated Canadian Caucasian patients with heart failure. Br J Clin Pharmacol 2008; 65(5):742–51.

[44] Sano H, Okamoto H, Kitabatake A, Iizuka K, Murakami T, Kawaguchi H. Increased mRNA expression of cardiac renin-angiotensin system and collagen synthesis in spontaneously hypertensive rats. Mol Cell Biochem 1998;178(1-2):51-8.

[45] Tiret L, Mallet C, Poirier O, Nicaud V, Millaire A, Bouhour JB et at. Lack of association between polymorphisms of eight candidate genes and idiopathic dilated cardiomyopathy: the CARDIGENE study. J Am Coll Cardiol 2000;35(1):29–35.

[46] Yamada Y, Ichihara S, Fujimura T, Yokota M.. Lack of association of polymorphisms of the angiotensin converting enzyme and angiotensinogen genes with nonfamilial hypertrophic or dilated cardiomyopathy. Am J Hypertens 1997;10(8):921–8.

[47] Takami S, Katsuya T, Rakugi H, Sato N, Nakata Y, Kamitani A et al. Angiotensin II Type 1 receptor gene polymorphism is associated with increase of left ventricular mass but not with hypertension. Am J Hypertens 1998;11(3 pt 1):316–21.

[48] Osterop Arthur PRM, Kofflard Marcel JM, Sandkuijl LA, Cate FJ ten, Krams R, Schalekamp Maarten ADH et al. AT1 Receptor A/C1166 Polymorphism Contributes to Cardiac Hypertrophy in Subjects With Hypertrophic Cardiomyopathy. Hypertension 1998;32(5):825-30.

[49] Broode O.E., Michel MC. (1999) Adrenergic and muscarinic receptor in the human heart. Pharmacol Rev 51: 651-689.

[50] Small KM, Rathz DA, Liggett BB. (2002) Identification of adrenergic receptor polymorphism.Method Enzymol 343: 459-475.

[51] Brodde O.E. (1988) The functional importance of beta1 and beta2 adrenoceptor in human heart. Am J cardiol 62: 24c-29c.

[52] Cohn JN, Levine TB, Olivari MT, Garberg V, Lura D. Francis GS et al. (1984) Plasma norepinephrine as a guide to prognosis in patients with chronic congestive heart failure. N Engl J Med 311: 819-823.

[53] Port JD, Bristow MR. (2001) Alerted beta-adrenergic receptor gene regulation and signaling in chronic heart failure. J Mol Cell Cardiol 33: 887-905.

[54] Kushwaha SS, Fallon JT, Fuster V. (1997) Restrictive cardiomyopathy. N Engl J Med 336(4):267-76.

[55] Forleoa C, Sorrentinoa S, Guidaa P, Romitob R, De Tommasia E, Iacovielloa M, Pitzalisc M. b1- and b2-adrenergic receptor polymorphisms affect susceptibility to idiopathic dilated cardiomyopathy. Journal of Cardiovascular Medicine 2007;8:589–95.

[56] Green SA, Cole G, Jacinto M, Innis M, Liggett SB. A polymorphism of the human beta 2-adrenergic receptor within the fourth transmembrane domain alters ligand binding and functional properties of the receptor. J Biol Chem 1993;268(31):23116-121.

[57] Green SA, Turki J, Innis M, Liggett SB. Amino-terminal polymorphisms of the human beta 2-adrenergic receptor impart distinct agonistpromoted regulatory properties. Biochemistry 1994;33(32):9414-19.

[58] Mason DA, Moore JD, Green SA, Liggett SB. A gain-of-function polymorphism in a G-protein coupling domain of the human beta1-adrenergic receptor. J Biol Chem 1999;274(18):12670-74.

[59] Rathz DA, Gregory KN, Fang Y, Brown KM, Liggett SB. Hierarchy of polymorphic variation and desensitization permutations relative to beta 1- and beta 2-adrenergic receptor signaling. J Biol Chem 2003;278(12):10784-89.

[60] Sandilands A, Yeo G, Brown MJ, O'Haughnessy KM. Functional responses of human beta1 adrenoceptors with defined haplotypes for the common 389R>G and 49S>G polymorphisms. Pharmacogenetics 2004;14(6):343-9.

[61] Bristow MR, Ginsburg R, Umans V, Fowler M, Minobe W, Rasmussen R et al. Beta 1- and beta 2-adrenergic-receptor subpopulations in nonfailing and failing human ventricular myocardium: coupling of both receptor subtypes to muscle contraction and selective beta 1-receptor downregulation in heart failure. Circ Res 1986;59(3):297–309.

[62] Turner AJ. Exploring the structure and function of zinc metallopeptidases: old enzymes and new discoveries. *Biochem Soc Trans* 2003;31:723–7.

[63] Turner AJ and Hooper NM. The angiotensin-converting enzyme gene family: genomics and pharmacology. *Trends Pharmacol Sci* 2002;23:177–183.

[64] Brosnihan KB, Neves LA, Joyner J, Averill DB, Chappell MC, Sarao R et al. Enhanced renal immunocytochemical expression of ANG(1–7) and ACE2 during pregnancy. Hypertension 2003;42:749–53.

[65] Burrell LM, Risvanis J, Kubota E, Dean RG, MacDonald PS, Lu S et al. Myocardial infarction increases ACE2 expression in rat and humans. Eur Heart J 2005;26:369–75.

[66] Donoghue M, Hsieh F, Baronas E, Godbout K, Gosselin M, Stagliano N et al. A novel angiotensin-converting enzyme-related carboxypeptidase (ACE2) converts angiotensin I to angiotensin 1–9. Circ Res 2000;87:E1–E9.

[67] Lely AT, Hamming I, van GH, Navis GJ. Renal ACE2 expression in human kidney disease. J Pathol 2004;204:587–93.

[68] Tikellis C, Johnston CI, Forbes JM, Burns WC, Thomas MC, Lew RA et al. Identification of angiotensin converting enzyme 2 in the rodent retina. Curr Eye Res 2004;29(6):419-27.

[69] Assayag P, Carre F, Chevalier B, Delcayre C, Mansier P, Swynghedauw B. Compensated cardiac hypertrophy: arrhythmogenicity and the new myocardial phenotype. I. Fibrosis. Cardiovasc Res 1997;34:439–44

[70] Lieb W, Graf J, Gotz A, Konig IR, Mayer B, Fischer M et al. Association of angiotensinconverting enzyme 2 (ACE2) gene polymorphisms with parameters of left ventricular hypertrophy in men. Results of the MONICA Augsburg echocardiographic substudy. J Mol Med 2006;84:88-96.

[71] Shu-xia W, Chun-yan FU, Yu-bao Z, Hu W, Yi S, Xi-qi XU et al. Polymorphisms of angiotensin-converting enzyme 2 gene associated with magnitude of left ventricular hypertrophy in male patients with hypertrophic cardiomyopathy. Chinese Medical Journal 2008;121:27-31.

[72] Poirier O, Nicaud V, McDonagh T, Dargie HJ, Desnos M, Dorent R et al. Polymorphisms of genes of the cardiac calcineurin pathway and cardiac hypertrophy. Eur J Hum Genet 2003;11:659–664.

[73] Chiu C, Tebo M, Ingles J, Yeates L, Arthur JW, Lind JM et al. Genetic screening of calcium regulation genes in familial hypertrophic cardiomyopathy. J Mol Cell Cardiol 2007;43:337–343.

[74] Friedrich F W, Bausero P, Sun Y, Treszl A, Kramer E, Juhr D et al . A new polymorphism in human calmodulin III gene promoter is a potential modifier gene for familial hypertrophic cardiomyopathy. Eur Heart J 2009;30:1648-55.

[75] Epstein ND. The molecular biology and pathophysiology of hypertrophic cardiomyopathy due to mutations in the beta myosin heavy chains and the essential and regulatory light chains. Adv Exp Med Biol 1998;453:105–14.

[76] Zhao Y, Meng XM, Wei YJ, Zhao XW, Liu D Q et al. Cloning and characterization of a novel cardiac-specific kinase that interacts specifically with cardiac troponin I. J Mol Med 2003;81:297–04.

[77] Wheeler FC, Tang H, Marks OA, Hadnott TN, Chu PL, Mao L et al . Tnni3k Modifies Disease Progression in Murine Models of Cardiomyopathy. PLoS Genet 2009;5:1000 -47.

[78] Lim DS, Lutucuta S, Bachireddy P, Youker K, Evans A, Entman M et al. Angiotensin II blockade reverses myocardial fibrosis in a transgenic mouse model of human hypertrophic cardiomyopathy. Circulation 2001;103(6):789–91.

[79] Shirani J, Pick R, Roberts WC, Maron BJ. Morphology and significance of the left ventricular collagen network in young patients with hypertrophic cardiomyopathy and sudden cardiac death. J Am Coll Cardiol 2000;35(1):36–44

4

Identification of Vulnerable Plaques with Optical Coherence Tomography

Takashi Kubo and Takashi Akasaka
Wakayama Medical University
Japan

1. Introduction

Recent advances in intravascular imaging have significantly improved the ability to detect high-risk, or vulnerable, plaque in vivo. Optical coherence tomography (OCT) is a new intravascular imaging method using a fiber-optic technology. The greatest advantage of OCT is its extraordinary high-resolution about 10-20 μm, which is approximately 10 times higher than that of intravascular ultrasound (IVUS). The high resolution afforded by this imaging modality is giving new insights into atherosclerotic plaque and the vascular responses after percutaneous coronary intervention (PCI). This report reviews the possibility of OCT for identification of vulnerable plaques in vivo.

2. Vulnerable plaque and pathology

The term "vulnerable plaque" is used to describe thrombosis prone plaques. Plaque rupture is the most frequent cause of coronary thrombosis, accounting for 60-65% for all coronary thrombi. The precursor lesion for plaque rupture is characterized by a thin fibrous cap heavily infiltrated macrophages and an underlying necrotic core. Virmani et al defined plaque vulnerability based on the actual thickness of the histological section from measurements made of plaque ruptures. The thin-cap fibroatheroma (TCFA) was defined as a lesion with a fibrous cap < 65 μm thick. A thickness of 65 μm was chosen as a criterion of instability because in rupture the mean cap thickness was 23 ± 19 μm; 95% of caps measured less than 65 μm within a limit of only two standard deviations. In addition to plaque rupture, plaque erosion can also result in coronary thrombosis. Erosion is usually found in the lesion with intimal thickening or thick-cap fibroatheroma. The thick fibrous cap in contrast to thin fibrous cap contains abundance of smooth muscle cells, proteoglycans and type III collagen but very few inflammatory cells.

3. Current OCT technology

OCT is an optical analogue of IVUS using near-infrared light. The wavelength used is 1,310 nm, which minimizes absorption of the light waves by water, protein, lipids, and hemoglobin without tissue damage. Based on the principles of low-coherence interferometry, the OCT system produces images with an axial resolution of 10-20 μm and a lateral resolution of 25-30 μm (Table 1). An optic probe, with dimensions similar to those of a coronary guide wire, delivers light to the tissue and collects the light reflected from the tissue. The image wire of current time-domain OCT system (M2/M3 TD-OCT imaging system, LightLab Imaging, Inc., Westford, Massachusetts) consists of a 0.006 inch (0.15 mm) fiber-optic core that rotates inside a sheath with a diameter of 0.016 inch (0.41 mm) (Figure 1). Because the near-infrared light signals are attenuated by red blood cells, OCT needs a blood-free imaging zone. To remove blood from the coronary artery and deliver the image wire, an over-the-wire occlusion balloon catheter is used. The diameter of the catheter shaft is 4.4 Fr and the balloon, designed for low-pressure inflation, was thin-walled polyurethane with a diameter of 3.8 mm at 0.3 atmospheres (< 8.5 mm at 1.0 atmospheres) and a length of 6.5 mm. Lactated Ringer's flushing solution is injected through the central inner lumen, which is shared with the image wire, and exits from the distal tip. The OCT imaging procedure starts with advancing the tip of a 0.014 inch (0.36 mm) coronary guide wire into the distal coronary artery. The occlusion catheter is then advanced over the wire until the balloon is positioned proximal to the target lesion. After the guide wire and OCT image wire are exchanged, lactated Ringer's solution is continuously flushed through the central lumen of the occlusion catheter by a power injector, and the balloon is inflated gradually by a custom inflation device until blood flow is fully occluded. Motorized pullback OCT imaging is performed at a rate of 1.0 mm/sec for a length of 30 mm. Images are acquired at 15 frames/sec and are digitally archived. The images are saved in the OCT imaging system console. During the procedure, electrocardiographic and hemodynamic features should be carefully monitored. Yamaguchi et al evaluated the safety and feasibility of OCT in 76 patients with coronary artery disease. Procedural success rates were 97%, and significant adverse cardiac events, including vessel dissection, acute myocardial infarction or fatal arrhythmia, were not observed. An inherent limitation of OCT is need for a blood-free imaging zone. The coronary occlusion for OCT image acquisition limits evaluation of left main or ostial coronary lesions. In addition, the time constraint imposed by blood flow interruption as well as slow frame rate of current OCT system prevents scanning of a significant length of a coronary artery during a single flush.

Recently, a second-generation OCT technology, termed Fourier-domain OCT (C7 FD-OCT imaging system, LightLab Imaging, Inc., Westford, Massachusetts), has been developed that solves the current time-domain OCT problems by imaging at much higher frame rates (100 frame/sec), a faster pullback speed (20 mm/sec), and a wider scan diameter (8.3mm) without loss of image quality (Table 2). These advantages result from the elimination of mechanical scanning of the reference mirror and signal-to-noise advantages of Fourier-domain signal processing (Figure 2). Imaging catheter of Fourier-domain OCT (Dragonfly Imaging Catheter, LightLab Imaging, Inc., Westford, Massachusetts), which is designed for rapid-exchange delivery, has 2.5-2.8 Fr crossing profile and can be delivered over a 0.014-inch guidewire through a 6 Fr or larger guide catheter. Injecting angiographic contrast media, or a mixture of commercially available dextran 40 and lactated Ringer's solution (low-molecular-weight Dextran L Injection, Otsuka Pharmaceutical Factory, Tokushima, Japan) through the guide catheter (4-6 ml/sec, 2-3 second) can achieve effective clearing of blood for Fourier-domain OCT imaging. The high frame rate and fast pullback speed of Fourier-domain OCT allows to image long coronary segments with minimal ischemia, eliminating the need for proximal vessel balloon occlusion during image acquisition.

	OCT	IVUS	Angioscopy	Angiography
Resolution (µm)	10-20	80-120	10-50	100-200
Probe size (mm)	0.016	0.7	0.8	n/a
Type of radiation	Near-IR light	Ultrasound	Visible light	X-ray
Other	Sub-surface tomogram	Sub-surface tomogram	Surface imaging only	Images of blood flow

Table 1. Comparison of the characteristics of coronary imaging methods.

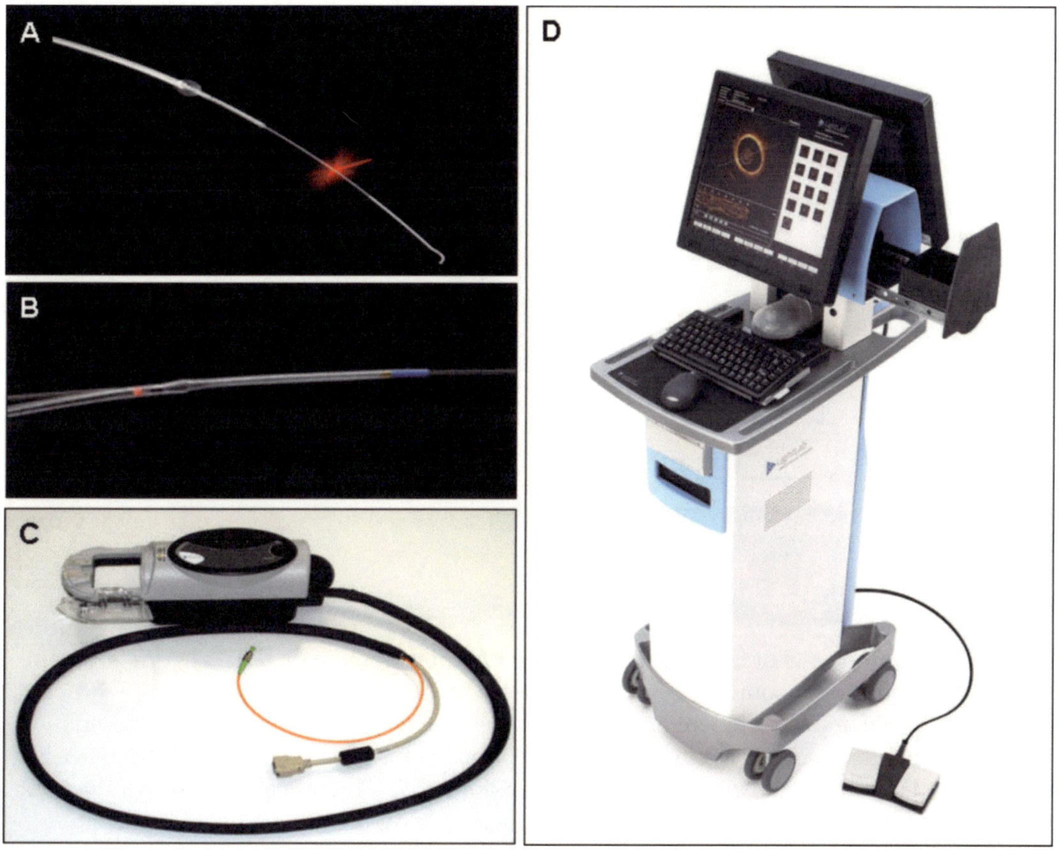

Fig. 1. LightLab OCT imaging system. (A) Time-domain OCT imaging wire. The time-domain OCT system employs a 0.016-inch fiber-optic imaging wire. (B) Fourier-domain OCT imaging catheter. Imaging catheter of Fourier-domain OCT has 2.5-2.8 Fr crossing profile and can be delivered over a 0.014-inch guidewire. (C) Patient interface unit. (D) OCT system console.

	Time-domain OCT	Fourier-domain OCT
Axial resolution (µm)	10-20	10-20
Lateral resolution (µm)	25-30	25-30
Scan diameter (mm)	6.8	8.3
Frame rate (f/sec)	15-20	100
Number of lines (/frame)	200-240	450
Maximum pullback speed (mm/sec)	2-3	20
Coronary occlusion for imaging	Required	Not required

Table 2. Performance of Fourier-domain OCT system in comparison with time-domain OCT System.

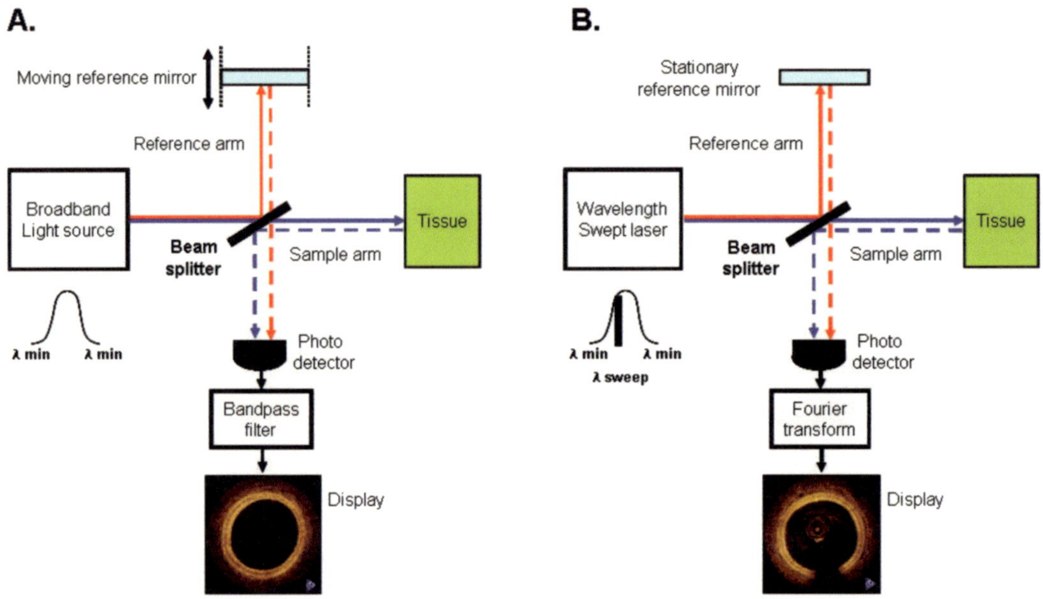

Fig. 2. Main components of time-domain OCT and Fourier-domain OCT. (A) In time-domain OCT, a broadband light source is divided by a beam splitter; part is sent to the tissue sample down the sample or measurement arm and the other down the reference arm to a moving mirror. The reflected signals are overlaid on a photo-detector. The intensity of interference is detected and used to create images. (B) In Fourier-domain OCT, the reference mirror does not move and the light source is a laser that sweeps its output rapidly over a broad band of wavelengths. Fourier transformation of the interference signals stored during a single sweep reconstructs the amplitude profile of the reflections, analogous to a single A-line in an ultrasound scan. Lasers with narrow line widths and wide sweep ranges enable the acquisition of Fourier-domain OCT images with high resolution over a wide range of depths.

4. Plaque characterization

Several histological examinations have demonstrated that OCT is highly sensitive and specific for plaque characterization. The high resolution of OCT allows us to identify 3-layer of coronary artery wall. In the OCT image, intima is observed as a signal rich layer nearest the lumen, media is visualized as a signal poor middle layer, and adventitia is identified as a signal-rich outer layer of artery wall (Figure 3). OCT enables more accurate estimation of the intimal thickness in comparison with IVUS which can not distinguish the boundary of the intima and media. Kume et al compared the coronary intima - media thickness and the intimal thickness of 54 coronary arterial segments evaluated by histological examination with the results of OCT and IVUS. There was a better agreement in intima - media thickness between OCT and histological examination than between IVUS and histological examination ($r=0.95$, $p<0.001$, mean difference = -0.01 ± 0.07 mm for OCT; $r=0.88$, $p<0.001$, mean difference = -0.03 ± 0.10 mm for IVUS). Moreover, there was an excellent agreement in the intimal thickness between OCT and histological examination ($r=0.98$, $p<0.001$, mean difference = 0.01 ± 0.04 mm).

Yabushita el al developed objective OCT image criteria for differentiating distinct components of atherosclerotic tissue. In their histology-controlled OCT study with 357 autopsy segments from 90 cadavers, fibrous plaques were characterized by homogeneous signal-rich regions (Figure 4), fibrocalcific plaques by signal-poor regions with sharp borders (Figure 5), and lipid-rich plaques by signal-poor regions with diffuse borders (Figure 6). Validation test revealed good intra- and inter-observer reliability (κ = 0.83–0.84) as well as excellent sensitivity and specificity—71-79% and 97-98% for fibrous plaques, 95-96% and 97% for fibrocalcific plaques, and 90-94% and 90-92% for lipid-rich plaques, respectively. These definitions have formed the basis of plaque composition interpretation (Table 3). Using these definitions, Kawasaki et al studied 128 coronary arterial sites from 42 coronary arteries of 17 cadavers by using OCT, integrated backscatter IVUS and conventional IVUS, and reported that OCT has a best potential for tissue characterization of coronary plaques (Fibrous tissue: sensitivity—98% vs. 94% vs. 93%, specificity—94% vs. 84% vs. 61%; Calcification: sensitivity—100% vs. 100% vs. 100%, specificity—100% vs. 99% vs. 99%; lipid pool: sensitivity—95% vs. 84% vs. 67%, specificity—98% vs. 97% vs. 95%). Kume et al also examined 166 sections from 108 coronary arterial segments of 40 consecutive human cadavers by using OCT and IVUS, and showed that OCT had a higher sensitivity for characterizing lipid-rich plaques than IVUS (85% vs. 59%, $p=0.030$). The intraobserver and interobserver agreement of OCT for characterizing plaque type was high ($\kappa=0.92$ and $\kappa=0.86$, respectively). These results suggest the possibility of OCT to identify vulnerable plaques which might contain lipid-rich necrotic core.

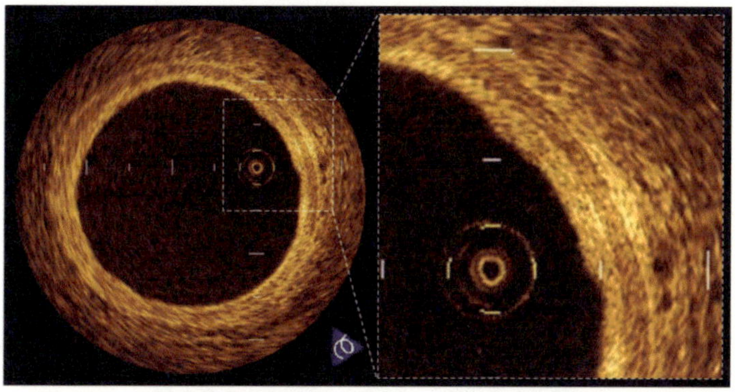

Fig. 3. Normal coronary wall. OCT image of normal coronary artery showing good contrast of the layers of the vessel wall including intima, media and adventitia.

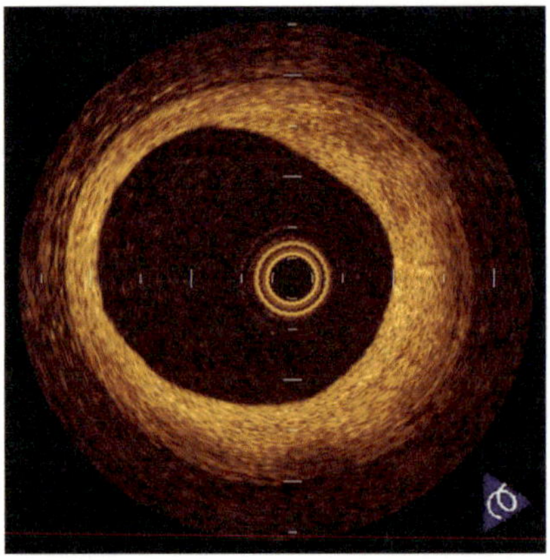

Fig. 4. Fibrous plaque. OCT image of a fibrous coronary plaque showing a homogeneous, signal-rich interior.

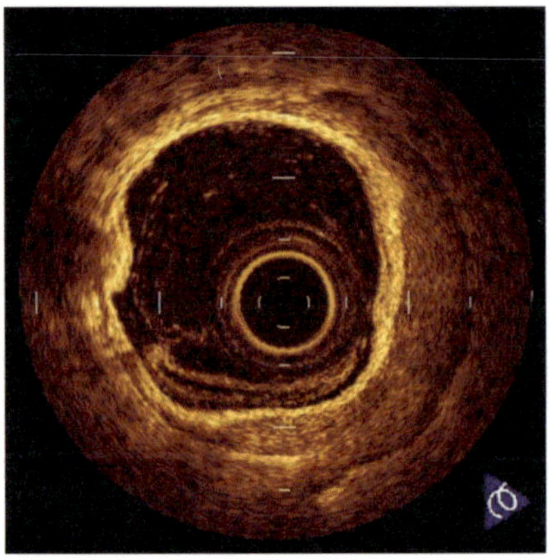

Fig. 5. Fibrocalcific plaque. OCT image of a fibrocalcific coronary plaque showing a sharply delineated region with a signal-poor interior.

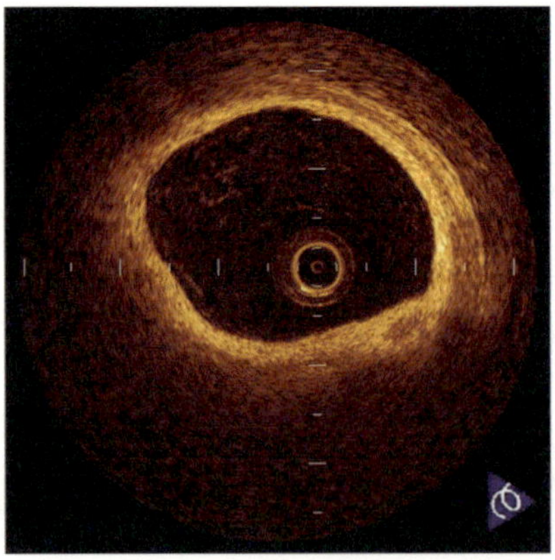

Fig. 6. Lipid-rich plaque. OCT image of a lipid-rich plaque showing a signal-poor lipid pool with poorly delineated borders beneath a homogeneous band, corresponding to fibrous cap.

Histology	OCT findings
Intima	Signal-rich layer near lumen
Media	Signal-poor layer in middle of artery wall
Adventitia	Signal-rich outer layer of artery wall
Fibrous tissue	Signal-rich, homogenous area
Calcium	Well-demarcated, heterogeneous area
Lipid	Signal-poor, poorly demarcated, homogenous area
Fibrous-cap	Signal-rich layer overlying signal-poor area

Table 3. OCT Characteristics of coronary microstructures

5. Vulnerable plaque detection

Since OCT has a near-histological grade resolution, many in-vitro and in vivo studies have been done to validate the capability of OCT to visualize vulnerable plaque features.

5.1 Plaque rupture and erosion

OCT can detect plaque rupture (Figure 7) and erosion (Figure 8) more precisely in comparison with conventional intravascular imaging techniques. Kubo et al used OCT, IVUS and angioscopy in patients with acute myocardial infarction (AMI) to assess the ability of each imaging method to detect the specific characteristics of vulnerable plaque. OCT was superior in detecting plaque rupture (73% vs. 40% vs. 43%, p=0.021), erosion (23% vs. 0% vs. 3%, p=0.003) and thrombus (100% vs. 33% vs. 100%, p<0.001) as compared with IVUS and angioscopy. Intra- and inter-observer variability of OCT yielded acceptable concordance for these characteristics (κ=0.61–0.83).

Using the capability of OCT for assessing plaque rupture and erosion in vivo, several studies have been performed to understand the mechanisms of acute coronary syndrome (ACS). Tanaka et al used OCT to investigate the relationship in patients with ACS between the morphology of a ruptured plaque and the patient's activity at the onset of ACS. Their data revealed that the thickness of the broken fibrous cap in the exertion group was significantly higher than in the rest-onset group (rest onset: 50 μm [interquartile median 15 μm]; exertion: 90 μm [interquartile median 65 μm], p<0.001), and some plaque rupture occurred in thick fibrous caps of > 65 μm depending on exertion levels. Mizukoshi et al used OCT to assess the relationship between clinical presentation and plaque morphologies in patients with unstable angina pectoris (UAP). In comparison with the Braunwald class I or II UAP patients, class III UAP patients had the highest frequency of plaque rupture (class I, 43%; class II, 13%; class III, 71%; p<0.001) and the thinnest fibrous cap (class I, median = 140 μm, quartile 1 to 3 = 90 to 160; class II, 150 μm, 120 to 160; class III, 60 μm, 40 to 105; p<0.001). In addition, class I UAP patients had the highest frequency of plaque erosion (class I, 32%; class II, 7%; class III, 8%; p=0.003) and the smallest minimum lumen area (class I, median 0.70 mm^2, quartiles 1 to 3 = 0.42 to 1.00; class II, 1.80 mm^2, 1.50 to 2.50; class III, 2.31 mm^2, 1.21 to 3.00; p<0.001). Recently, Ino et al used OCT to investigate the difference of culprit lesion morphologies between ST-segment elevation myocardial infraction (STEMI) and non–ST-segment elevation ACS (NSTEACS). The incidence of plaque rupture was significantly higher in STEMI compared with NSTEACS (70% vs. 47%, p=0.033). Although the lumen area at the site of plaque rupture was similar in the both groups, the area of ruptured cavity was significantly larger in STEMI compared with NSTEACS (2.52 ± 1.36

mm^2 vs. 1.67 ± 1.37 mm^2, p=0.034). Furthermore, the ruptured plaque of which aperture was open-wide against the direction of coronary flow was more often seen in STEMI compared with NSTEACS (46% vs. 17%, p=0.036).

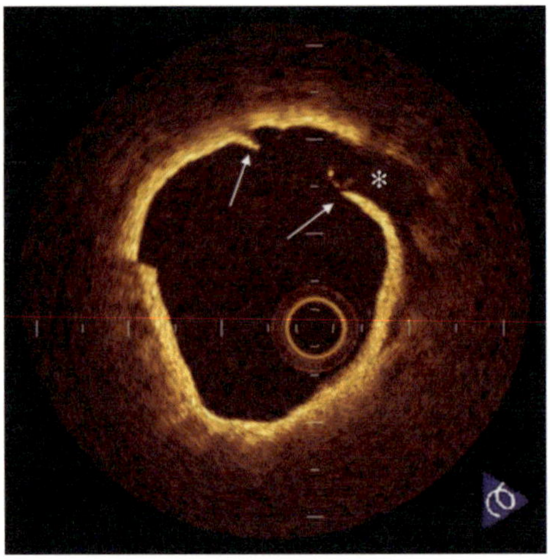

Fig. 7. Plaque rupture. Plaque rupture is defined as the presence of fibrous-cap discontinuity (arrows) and a cavity formation (*) in the plaque.

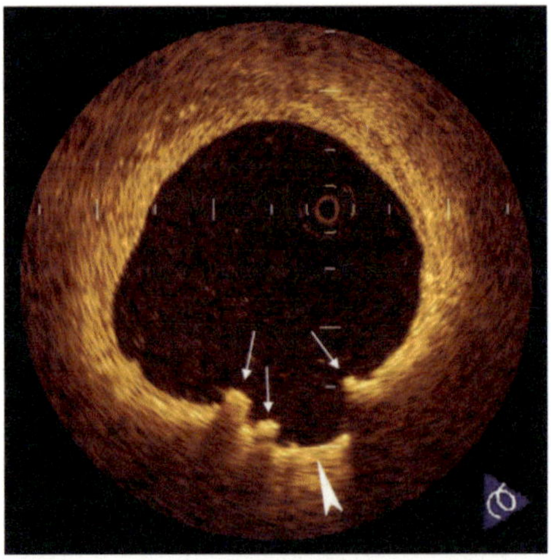

Fig. 8. Plaque erosion. Erosion (arrowhead) is usually comprised of OCT evidence of thrombi (arrows), an irregular luminal surface, and no evidence of cap rupture evaluated in multiple adjacent frames.

5.2 Thin-cap fibroatheroma

OCT might be the best tool available to detect TCFAs in vivo (Figure 9). Kume et al examined the reliability of OCT for measuring the fibrous cap thickness. In the examination of 35 lipid-rich plaques from 38 human cadavers, there was a good correlation of the fibrous cap thickness between OCT and histological examination (r = 0.90; p<0.001). In the clinical setting, Sawada et al compared the feasibility for detecting TCFA between OCT and virtual histology IVUS. Although the positive ratio of virtual histology IVUS for detecting TCFA was 45.9%, that of OCT was 77.8%. Jang et al analyzed OCT images among 57 patients who presented with stable angina pectoris (SAP), ACS, or AMI. The AMI group was more likely than the ACS group, who was more likely than the SAP group, to have a thinner cap, more lipid, and a higher percentage of TCFA (72% vs. 50% vs. 20%, respectively, $p = 0.012$). On top of its reliability as a tool to measure the fibrous-cap thickness in vivo, a recent OCT study conducted by Takarada et al demonstrated that the lipid-lowering therapy with statin for 9 months follow-up significantly increased the fibrous-cap thickness in patients with hypercholesterolemia (151 ± 110 to 280 ± 120 µm, $p<0.01$). As therapies to prevent or make regression of atherosclerosis are developed, OCT can help to assess the treatment efficacy.

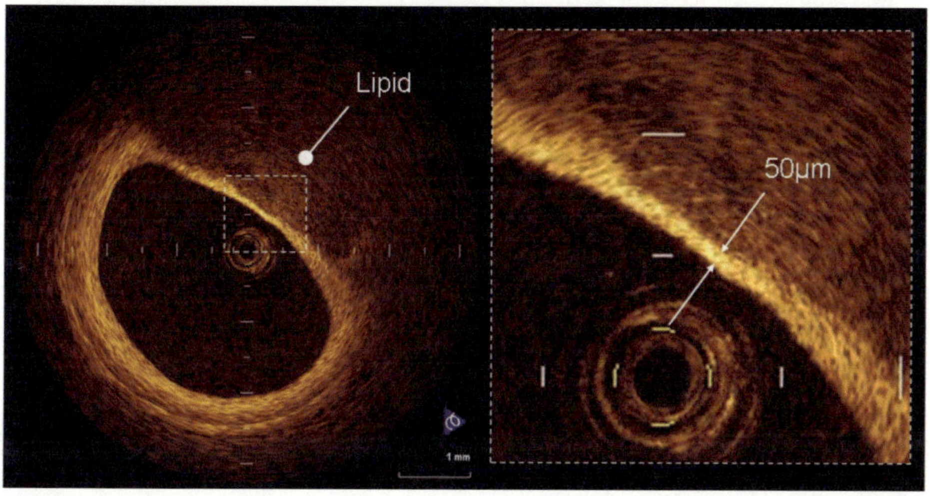

Fig. 9. Thin-cap fibroatheroma. A fibrous cap is identified as a signal-rich homogenous region overlying a lipid core, which is characterized by a signal-poor region in the OCT image. Thin-cap fibroatheroma is defined as a plaque with a fibrous cap measuring <65 µm.

5.3 Thrombus

The OCT characteristics of coronary thrombi were studied by Kume et al in 108 coronary arterial segments at postmortem examination. Red thrombus (Figure 10-A), which mainly consists of red-blood cell, is identified as high-backscattering protrusions inside the lumen of the artery with signal-free shadow, while white thrombus (Figure 10-B), which mainly consists of platelet and fibrin, is identified as signal-rich, low-backscattering protrusions in the OCT image. Using a measurement of the OCT signal attenuation within the thrombus, the authors demonstrated that a cut-off value of 250 µm in the 1/2 width of signal attenuation can differentiate white from red thrombi with a high sensitivity (90%) and specificity (88%).

5.4 Plaque neovascularization

Plaque neovascularization is a common feature of vulnerable plaque. Proliferation of micro-vessels is considered to be related with intraplaque haemorrhage and plaque destabilization. The high resolution of OCT provides an opportunity to detect plaque neovascularization in vivo (Figure 11). Kitabata et al demonstrated increase of micro-vessels density in TCFAs by using OCT. The presence of micro-vessels in the plaques was also associated with positive vessel remodeling and elevated hs-CRP levels. The OCT evaluation of micro-vessels density might be helpful to assess plaque vulnerability.

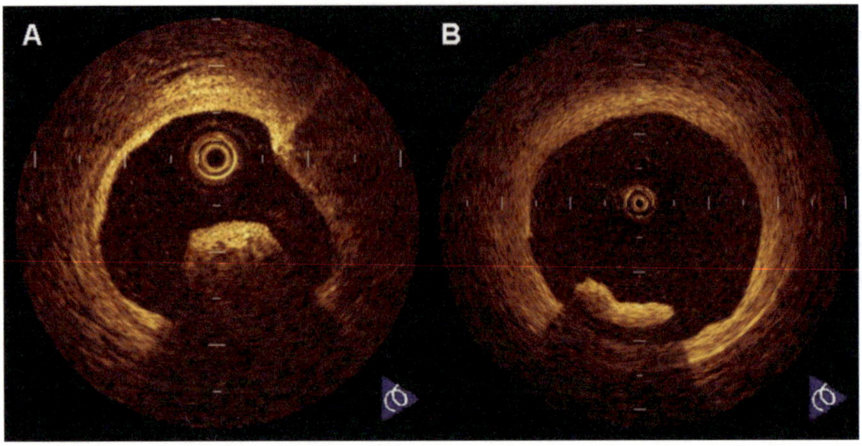

Fig. 10. Intracoronary thrombi. (A) Red thrombus is defined as a protrusion inside the lumen of the artery with high signal attenuation in the OCT image. (B) White thrombus is defined as a protruding mass with low signal attenuation in the OCT image.

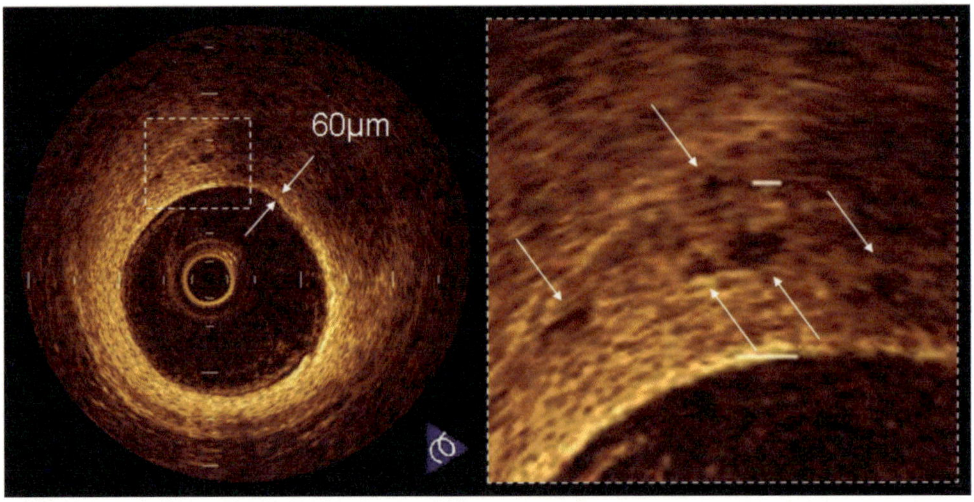

Fig. 11. Micro-vessels in the coronary plaque. Vessels within the intima (arrows) appear as signal poor voids that are sharply delineated.

5.5 Macrophages

A unique aspect of OCT is its ability to visualize the macrophages (Figure 12). Tearney et al proposed the potential of OCT to assess macrophage distribution within fibrous caps. There was a high degree of positive correlation between OCT and histological measurements of fibrous cap macrophage density ($r<0.84$, $P<0.001$). A range of OCT signal standard deviation thresholds (6.15% to 6.35%) yielded 100% sensitivity and specificity for identifying caps containing >10% CD68 staining.

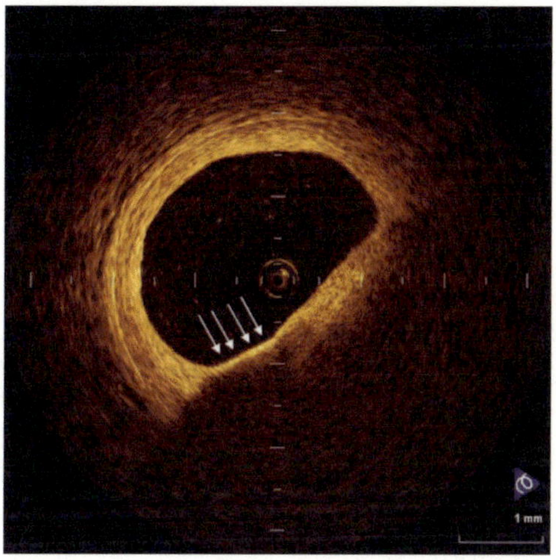

Fig. 12. Macrophage. Macrophages (arrows) are seen as signal-rich, distinct or confluent punctuate regions that exceed the intensity of background speckle noise.

6. Multiple lesion instability

In the diffuse nature of coronary atherosclerosis, plaque instability might be expected to develop in a multifocal pattern. Virmani et al showed that 70% of cases of sudden cardiac death had non-ruptured TCFAs. Most non-ruptured TCFAs and ruptured plaque are localized in the proximal 1/3 of the major coronary arteries. In a 3-vessel VH-IVUS study, Hong et al demonstrated that 72% of patients with AMI or UAP had multiple VH-IVUS-derived TCFAs. Asakura et al performed 3-vessel angioscopic examination in AMI and showed that yellow plaques were equally prevalent in the infarct-related and non-infarct-related coronary arteries. In the multifocal OCT study, Tanaka et al reported that 7% of patients with acute coronary syndrome had >2 OCT-derived TCFAs in the entire culprit coronary artery. Kubo et al evaluated non-culprit vessels by using OCT and demonstrated a greater frequency of multiple OCT-derived TCFAs in AMI patients than in SAP patients. Fujii et al performed a prospective OCT analysis of all 3 major coronary arteries to evaluate the incidence and predictors of TCFAs in patients with AMI and SAP. Multiple TCFAs were observed more frequently in AMI patients than in SAP patients (69% vs. 10%, $p<0.001$). In the entire cohort, multivariate analysis revealed that the only independent predictor of TCFA was AMI (OR=4.12, 95% CI=2.35-9.87, p=0.020,). These OCT results support the theory that acute coronary syndrome is a multifocal process (Figure 13).

7. Drug-eluting stent in vulnerable lesion

Drug-eluting stent has been reported to impair local vascular healing with delayed endothelization. The patients with ACS present a higher risk for thrombotic complication after stent implantation in comparison with SAP. Therefore, vascular response after drug-eluting stent implantation in the vulnerable lesion is a great concern. Recently, Kubo et al used OCT to evaluate lesion morphologies after drug-eluting stent implantation in the

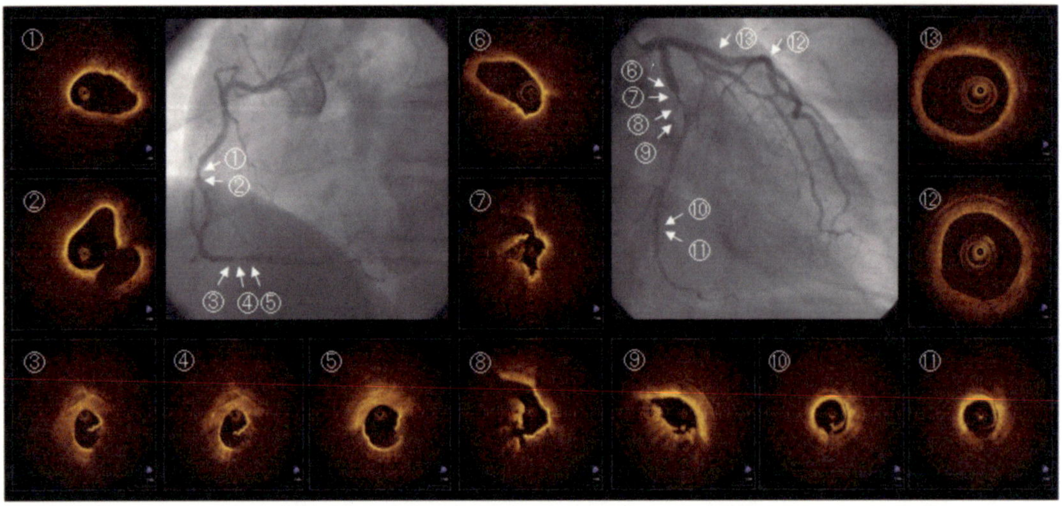

Fig. 13. Multiple lesion instability in patient with acute myocardial infarction. Coronary angiogram showed that the culprit lesion was located in the proximal site of left circumflex coronary artery (diameter stentosis = 99%; TIMI-II flow). Thin-cap fibroatheroma (⑥), plaque rupture (⑦, ⑧) and intracoronary thrombi (⑦, ⑧) were observed at the culprit lesion by OCT. Although the plaques in left descending coronary artery (⑫, ⑬) were not unstable, thin-cap fibroatheroma (①-⑤) and plaque rupture (③, ④, ⑤, ⑩, ⑪) was detected by OCT in the non-culprit lesions of right coronary artery and distal left circumflex coronary artery.

unstable lesions. Inadequate stent apposition (67% vs. 32%, p=0.038) and tissue protrusion (79% vs. 42%, p=0.005) after PCI were observed more frequently in UAP patients compared with SAP patients. Plaque rupture was significantly increased after PCI in UAP patients (42% to 75%, p=0.018). The persistence of core cavity after plaque rupture at 9 months' follow-up (Figure 14) was observed more frequently in UAP patients compared with SAP patients (28% vs. 4%, p=0.031). At 9 months' follow-up, the incidence of inadequately apposed stent (33% vs. 4%, p=0.012) and partially uncovered stent by neointima (72% vs. 37%, p=0.019) was significantly greater in UAP patients than that in SAP patients. Residual plaque rupture behind the stent and uncovered stent struts might be important risks for late stent thrombosis because the lipid content of exposed necrotic core and metal stent is highly thrombogenic (Figure 14). Although arterial healing with excessive neointimal growth leads to restenosis, neointima (or endothelium) that seals the underlying thrombogenic components may protect against late stent thrombosis.

8. Atherosclerotic changes in neointimal tissue inside stent

Atherosclerotic changes and consequent plaque vulnerability occur in the neointimal tissue inside the stent. Takano et al observed the neointimal characteristics of bare-metal stents in early phase (<6 months) and late phase (> 5 years) by using OCT. Lipid-rich neointima was often seen in the late phase compared with the early phase (67% vs. 0%, p<0.001). The appearance of intraintima neovascularization was more prevalent in the late phase than the early phase (62% vs. 0%, p<0.001). Kashiwagi et al used OCT to examine the stented segments in cases with very late stent thrombosis, and reported neointimal plaque rupture. Atherosclerotic progression in neointimal tissue inside the stents might contribute to late clinical events after stent treatment (Figure 15).

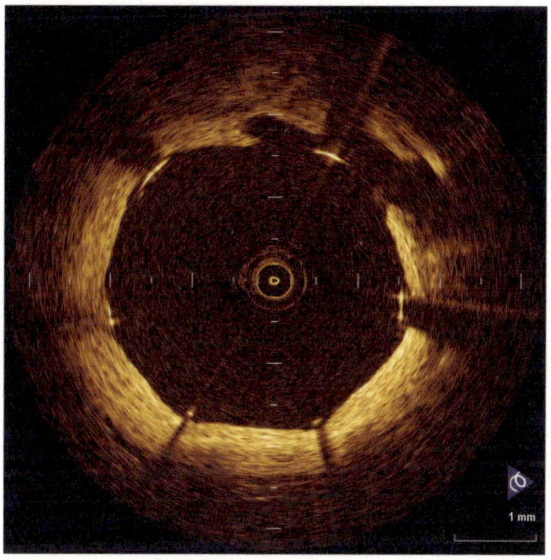

Fig. 14. Residual plaque rupture behind coronary stent. The OCT image at 9-month follow-up after drug-eluting stent implantation shows persistence of core cavity and inadequately-apposed stent struts without neointimal coverage.

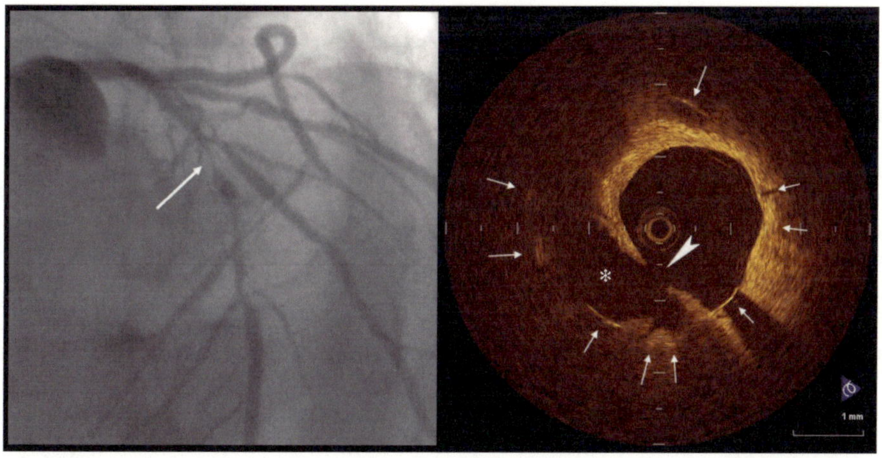

Fig. 15. A case with neointimal plaque rupture inside bare-metal stent. A 60-year-old man was given a diagnosis of stable angina and treated with a bare-metal stent (3.5 x 18 mm) deployed to the mid-portion of the left anterior descending artery 8 years ago. A follow-up coronary angiography at 6 months after the procedure presented no restenosis. Eight years after stent deployment, he suddenly suffered recurrence of angina and was admitted to the hospital. A coronary angiography showed severe in-stent restenosis of the previously stented segment of the LAD (arrow). Before any interventions, OCT was performed. OCT clearly revealed plaque rupture (arrowhead) and cavity formation (*) within well expanded stent struts (arrows).

9. Limitations

OCT has a relatively shallow axial penetration depth of 2mm. The OCT signal does not reach the back wall of thick atherosclerotic lesions. The penetration depth of OCT depends on tissue characteristics. Lipid-rich plaque or coronary thrombus causes OCT signal attenuation, which interrupts to observe deep layers of coronary artery wall. OCT is not appropriate for the visualization of whole vessel and the evaluation of arterial remodeling.

10. Current technology challenges

Recently, Tearney et al reported that Fourier-domain OCT, called optical frequency-domain imaging by author's group, enables imaging of the 3-dimensional microstructure of long segments of coronary arteries. In addition, Fourier-domain OCT facilitates the acquisition of spectroscopic and polarization, Doppler and other imaging modes for plaque characterization. When Fourier-domain OCT is fully exploited, it has the potential to dramatically change the way that physicians and researchers understand the coronary artery disease in order to better diagnose and treat disease.

11. Conclusion

The high resolution of OCT provides histology-grade definition of the microstructure of coronary plaque in vivo. OCT allows a greater understanding of the pathophysiology of vulnerable plaque. Whether OCT will have an established clinical role in vulnerable plaque detection must depend on the outcomes of future prospective natural history studies. Precise identification of thrombosis-prone vulnerable plaque could change our approach to the treatment of coronary atherosclerotic disease and contribute to prevention of ACS.

12. Acknowledgment

The authors thank Teruyoshi Kume, MD; Hironori Kitabata, MD; Yasushi Ino, MD; Takashi Tanimoto, MD; Kohei Ishibashi, MD; Yoshiki Matsuo, MD; Yasushi Okumoto, MD for assistance with OCT image acquisition and analysis.

13. References

Akasaka, T.; Kubo, T. & Mizukoshi, M. (2010). Pathophysiology of acute coronary syndrome assessed by optical coherence tomography. *J Cardiol*, Vol. 56, No.1, (July), pp. 8-14

Ino, Y.; Kubo, T. & Tanaka, A. (2011). Difference of culprit lesion morphologies between ST-segment elevation myocardial infarction and non-ST-segment elevation acute coronary syndrome: an optical coherence tomography study. *JACC Cardiovasc Interv*, Vol. 4, No.1, (January), pp. 76-82

Fujii, K.; Masutani. M. & Okumura, T. (2008). Frequency and predictor of coronary thin-cap fibroatheroma in patients with acute myocardial infarction and stable angina pectoris a 3-vessel optical coherence tomography study. *J Am Coll Cardiol*, Vol. 52, No.9, (August 26), pp. 787-788

Gonzalo, N.; Serruys, PW. & Okamura, T. (2009). Optical coherence tomography patterns of stent restenosis. *Am Heart J*, Vol. 158, No. 2, (August), pp. 284-293

Guagliumi, G.; Costa, MA. & Sirbu, V. (2011). Strut coverage and late malapposition with paclitaxel-eluting stents compared with bare metal stents in acute myocardial infarction: optical coherence tomography substudy of the Harmonizing Outcomes with Revascularization and Stents in Acute Myocardial Infarction (HORIZONS-AMI) Trial. *Circulation*, Vol. 123, No. 3, (January 25), pp. 274-281

Habara, M.; Terashima, M. & Nasu, K. (2011). Difference of tissue characteristics between early and very late restenosis lesions after bare-metal stent implantation: an optical coherence tomography study. *Circ Cardiovasc Interv*, Vo. 4, No. 3, (June), pp. 232-238

Jang, IK.; Tearney, GJ. & MacNeill, B. (2005). In vivo characterization of coronary atherosclerotic plaque by use of optical coherence tomography. *Circulation*, Vol. 111, No.12, (March 29), pp. 1551-1555

Kashiwagi, M.; Tanaka, A. & Kitabata, H. (2009). Relationship between coronary arterial remodeling, fibrous cap thickness and high-sensitivity C-reactive protein levels in patients with acute coronary syndrome. *Circ J*, Vol. 73, No.7, (July), pp. 1291-1295

Kashiwagi, M.; Tanaka, A. & Kitabata, H. (2009). Feasibility of noninvasive assessment of thin-cap fibroatheroma by multidetector computed tomography. *JACC Cardiovasc Imaging*, Vol. 2, No.12, (Descember), pp. 1412-1419

Kashiwagi, M.; Kitabata, H. & Tanaka, A. (2010). Very late clinical cardiac event after BMS implantation: in vivo optical coherence tomography examination. *JACC Cardiovasc Imaging*, Vol. 3, No.5, (May), pp. 525-527.

Kawasaki, M.; Bouma, BE. & Bressner, J. (2006). Diagnostic Accuracy of Optical Coherence Tom ography and Integrated Backscatter Intravascular Ultrasound Images for Tissue Characterization of Human Coronary Plaques. *J Am Coll Cardiol*, Vol. 48, No.1, (July 4), pp. 81-88

Kataiwa, H.; Tanaka, A. & Kitabata, H. (2008). Safety and usefulness of non-occlusion image acquisition technique for optical coherence tomography. *Circ J*, Vol. 72, No.9, (September), pp. 1536-1537

Kitabata, H.; Kubo, T. & Akasaka, T. (2008) Identification of multiple plaque ruptures by optical coherence tomography in a patient with acute myocardial infarction: a three-vessel study. *Heart*. Vol. 94, No.5, (May), pp. 544

Kitabata, H.; Tanaka, A. & Kubo, T. (2010). Relation of microchannel structure identified by optical coherence tomography to plaque vulnerability in patients with coronary artery disease. *Am J Cardiol*, Vol. 105, No.12, (Jun 15), pp. 1673-1678

Kubo, T.; Imanishi, T. & Takarada, S. (2007). Assessment of culprit lesion morphology in acute myocardial infarction: ability of optical coherence tomography compared with intravascular ultrasound and coronary angioscopy. *J Am Coll Cardiol*, Vol. 50, No.10, (September 4), pp. 933-939

Kubo, T.; Imanishi, T. & Takarada, S. (2008). Implication of plaque color classification for assessing plaque vulnerability: A coronary angioscopy and optical coherence tomography investigation. *JACC Cardiovasc Interv*. Vol. 1, No.1, (February), pp. 74-80.

Kubo, T.; Imanishi, T. & Takarada, S. (2008). Comparison of vascular response after sirolimus-eluting stent implantation between unstable angina pectoris and stable angina pectoris: a serial optical coherence tomography study. *JACC Cardiovasc Imaging*, Vol. 1, No.4, (July), pp. 475-484

Kubo, T. & Akasaka, T. (2009). Reply Letter to: Optical coherence tomography to diagnose under-expansion of a drug eluting stent. *JACC Cardiovasc Imaging*, Vol. 2, No.2, (February), pp. 246

Kubo, T. & Akasaka, T. (2008). Recent advances in intracoronary imaging techniques: focus on optical coherence tomography. *Expert Review of Medical Devices*, Vol.5, No.6, (November), pp. 691-697

Kubo, T.; Imanishi, T. & Kashiwagi, M. (2010). Multiple coronary lesion instability in patients with acute myocardial infarction as determined by optical coherence tomography. *Am J Cardiol*, Vol.105, No.3, (February), pp. 318-322

Kubo, T.; Xu, C. & Wang, Z. (2011). Plaque and Thrombus evaluation by Optical Coherence Tomography. *Int J Cardiovasc Imaging*, Vol. 27, No. 2, (February), pp. 289-298

Kubo, T.; Nakamura, N. & Matsuo, Y. (2011). Virtual histology intravascular ultrasound compared with optical coherence tomography for identification of thin-cap fibroatheroma. *Int Heart J*, Vol. 52, No. 3, (May), pp. 175-179

Kume, T; Akasaka, T. & Kawamoto, T. (2005). Assessment of coronary intima-media thickness by optical coherence tomography: comparison with intravascular ultrasound. *Circ J*, Vol. 69, No.8, (August), pp. 903-907

Kume, T; Akasaka, T. & Kawamoto, T. (2006). Assessment of Coronary Arterial Plaque by Optical Coherence Tomography. *Am J Cardiol*, Vol. 97, No.8, (April), pp. 1172-1175

Kume, T.; Akasaka, T. & Kawamoto, T. (2006). Assessment of coronary arterial thrombus by optical coherence tomography. *Am J Cardiol*, Vol. 97, No.2, (June), pp. 1713-1717

Kume, T.; Akasaka, T. & Kawamoto, T. (2006). Measurement of the thickness of the fibrous cap by optical coherence tomography. *Am Heart J*, Vol. 152, No.4, (October),pp. e1-4

Kume, T.; Okura, H. & Yamada, R. (2009). Frequency and spatial distribution of thin-cap fibroatheroma assessed by 3-vessel intravascular ultrasound and optical coherence tomography. *Circ J*, Vol. 73, No.6, (June), pp. 1086-1091

Liu, Y.; Imanishi, T. & Kubo, T. (2010). Assessment by optical coherence tomography of stent struts across side branch. -Comparison of bare-metal stents and drug-elution stents. *Circ J*, Vol. 75, No.1, (Descember 24), pp. 106-112

MacNeill, BD.; Jang, IK. & Bouma, BE. (2004). Focal and multi-focal plaque macrophage distributions in patients with acute and stable presentations of coronary artery disease. *J Am Coll Cardiol*, Vol. 44, No. 5, (September 1), pp. 972-979

Mizukoshi, M. Imanishi, T. & Tanaka, A. (2010). Clinical classification and plaque morphology determined by optical coherence tomography in unstable angina pectoris. *Am J Cardiol*, Vol. 106, No.3, (August), pp. 323-328

Nadkarni, SK.; Pierce, MC. & Park, BH. (2007). Measurement of collagen and smooth muscle cell content in atherosclerotic plaques using polarization-sensitive optical coherence tomography. *J Am Coll Cardiol*, Vol. 49, No.13, (April), pp. 1474-1481

Nishiguchi, T.; Kitabata, H. & Tanaka, A. (2010). Very late stent thrombosis after drug-eluting stent in segment with neointimal tissue coverage. *JACC Cardiovasc Imaging*, Vol. 3, No.4, (April), pp. 445-446

Prati, F.; Regar, E. & Mintz, GS. (2010). Expert review document on methodology, terminology, and clinical applications of optical coherence tomography: physical principles, methodology of image acquisition, and clinical application for assessment of coronary arteries and atherosclerosis. *Eur Heart J*, Vol. 31, No. 4, (February), pp. 401-415

Raffel, OC.; Akasaka, T. & Jang, IK. (2008). Cardiac optical coherence tomography. *Heart,* Vol.94, No.9, (September), pp. 1200-1210

Sawada, T.; Shite, J. & Garcia-Garcia, HM. (2008). Feasibility of combined use of intravascular ultrasound radiofrequency data analysis and optical coherence tomography for detecting thin-cap fibroatheroma. *Eur Heart J,* Vol. 29, No. 9, (May), pp. 1136-1146

Stary, HC. (2000). Natural history and histological classification of atherosclerotic lesions: an update. *Arterioscler Thromb Vasc Biol,* Vol. 20, No. 5, (May), pp. 1177-1178

Takano, M.; Yamamoto, M. & Inami, S. (2009). Appearance of lipid-laden intima and neovascularization after implantation of bare-metal stents extended late-phase observation by intracoronary optical coherence tomography. *J Am Coll Cardiol,* Vol. 55, No. 1, (December), pp. 26-32

Takarada, S.; Imanishi, T. & Kubo, T. (2009). Effect of statin therapy on coronary fibrous-cap thickness in patients with acute coronary syndrome: Assessment by optical coherence tomography study. *Atherosclerosis,* Vol. 202, No.2, (February), pp. 491-497

Takarada, S.; Imanishi, T. & Liu, Y. (2010). Advantage of next-generation frequency-domain optical coherence tomography compared with conventional time-domain system in the assessment of coronary lesion. *Catheter Cardiovasc Interv,* Vol. 75, No.2, (February 1), pp. 202-206

Takarada, S.; Imanishi, T. & Ishibashi, K. (2010). The effect of lipid and inflammatory profiles on the morphological changes of lipid-rich plaques in patients with non-ST-segment elevated acute coronary syndrome: follow-up study by optical coherence tomography and intravascular ultrasound. *JACC Cardiovasc Interv,* Vol. 3, No.7, (July), pp. 766-772

Tanaka, A.; Imanishi, T. & Kitabata, H. (2008). Distribution and frequency of thin-capped fibroatheromas and ruptured plaques in the entire culprit coronary artery in patients with acute coronary syndrome as determined by optical coherence tomography. *Am J Cardiol,* Vol. 102, No.8, (October 15), pp. 975-979

Tanaka, A.; Imanishi, T. & Kitabata, H. (2008). Morphology of exertion-triggered plaque rupture in patients with acute coronary syndrome: an optical coherence tomography study. *Circulation,* Vol. 118, No.23, (December 2), pp. 2368-2373

Tanaka, A.; Imanishi, T. & Kitabata, H. (2009). Lipid-rich plaque and myocardial perfusion after successful stenting in patients with non-ST-segment elevation acute coronary syndrome: an optical coherence tomography study. *Eur Heart J,* Vol. 30, No.11, (June), pp. 1348-1355

Tanimoto, T.; Imanishi, T. & Tanaka, A. (2009). Various types of plaque disruption in a culprit coronary artery visualized by optical coherence tomography in a patient with unstable angina. *Circ J,* Vol. 73, No.1, (January), pp. 187-189

Tearney, GJ.; Yabushita, H. & Houser, SL. (2003). Quantification of macrophage content in atherosclerotic plaques by optical coherence tomography. *Circulation,* Vol. 107, No.1, (January), pp. 113-119

Tearney, GJ.; Waxman, S. & Shishkov, M. (2008). Three-dimensional coronary artery microscopy by intracoronary optical frequency domain imaging. *JACC Cardiovasc Imaging,* Vol. 1, No.6, (November), pp. 752-761

Virmani, R.; Kolodgie, FD. & Burke, AP. (2000). Lessons from sudden coronary death: a comprehensive morphological classification scheme for atherosclerotic lesions. *Arterioscler Thromb Vasc Biol*, Vol. 20, No. 5, (May), pp. 1262-1275

Virmani, R.; Burke, AP. & Kolodgie, FD. (2003). Pathology of the thin-cap fibroatheroma: a type of vulnerable plaque. *J Interv Cardiol*, Vol. 16, No. 3, (June), pp. 267-272

Yabushita, H.; Bouma, BE. & Houser, SL. (2002). Characterization of human atherosclerosis by optical coherence tomography. *Circulation,* Vol. 106, No.13, (September), pp. 1640-1645

Yamaguchi, T.; Terashima, M. & Akasaka, T. (2008). Safety and feasibility of an intravascular optical coherence tomography image wire system in the clinical setting. *Am J Cardiol,* Vol. 101, No.5, (March), pp. 562-567

Part 3

Specific Therapy

5

Coronary Artery Disease in the Elderly

Milton Alcaíno and Denisse Lama
Cardiology Department, Hospital Dipreca, Santiago
Chile

1. Introduction

Cardiovascular (CV) disease is the most frequent diagnosis in elderly people and it is the leading cause of death in both men and women older than 65 years of age. The high morbidity and mortality from cardiovascular disease warrant aggressive approaches to prevention and treatment that have been shown to be effective in older patients. Increased emphasis is being placed on preventive strategies for cardiovascular disease the elderly and improving the quality of care using therapies that were not designed for them. Historically physicians are prone to more conservative and use less aggressive therapies. Nevertheless, given their high-risk status, the elderly with heart disease are also a group that is very likely to experience improvements in clinical outcomes and functional status with revascularization. However, they are also more likely to experience procedural complications, owing to age-related physiological changes, frailty, and comorbidities. As such, the decision on when to pursue revascularization in elderly patients, and if so, how to revascularize, is complex.

The limited representation of elderly patients in clinical trials has resulted in fewer data about the effectiveness of various strategies in this population. Moreover, the atypical clinical presentations of coronary artery disease (CAD) in elderly patients, and the consequent difficulty in diagnosis, have resulted in suboptimal implementation of treatment and secondary preventive measures by health care professionals. Increased investigation at both the basic level and clinical level is necessary to identify therapies that will benefit older patients on the basis of both the pathophysiology of age-related CV disease and the frequent presence of comorbid diseases.

It is important to assess the risk of the patient individually to provide the best treatment strategy. Decisions regarding medical therapy versus revascularization; PCI or CABG should be based not only on symptoms, severity of CAD, left ventricular function but in the context of other comorbidities, lifestyle, projected life span, and preferences. In hospitals without PCI capability reperfusion therapy with thrombolytic should be considered, regarding thrombolytic drugs especially in very old patients, streptokinase should be considered.

The purpose of this chapter is to explain the therapeutic approaches and considerations that must be taken when dealing with an elderly patient with CAD. To illustrate this we reviewed bibliographic databases such as medline and pubmed, with key words coronary artery disease, revascularization, thombolysis, coronary percutaneus intervention and elderly for our search.

Finally, we will demonstrate our experience in Chile with one of the few clinical trials in our country that includes the elderly as their main subjects of study, comparing different approaches of treatment towards CAD in this specific group of patients.

2. Epidemiology

The worldwide population of people 65 years of age and older are projected to increase to 973 million or 12 percent by 2030 and to 20 percent of the population by 2050. Most definitions of elderly are based on chronological age. The World Health Organization uses 60 years of age to define elderly whereas most classifications use the age of 65 years, but patients older than 75 years are more fragile.

Cardiovascular disease is the most important cause of death in both men and women in this age group. More than 80 percent of all deaths attributable to cardiovascular diseases occur in people older than 65 years with approximately 60 percent of deaths in patients older than 75 years old. High blood pressure, heart failure with preserved systolic function and multivessel disease are very common. Systolic blood pressure increases with aging, it occurs in one half to two thirds of people older than 65 years of age, and heart failure (HF) is the most frequent hospital discharge diagnosis among older patients. In addition, cardiovascular disease in the elderly usually is associated with other medical conditions given that eighty percent of people over 65 years old have at least one chronic medical condition, and half have at least two.

The prevalence and severity of CAD increases with age in both men and women. A significant number of people older than the age of 60 years have significant CAD with increasing prevalence of left main or triple-vessel disease. Evidence of myocardial infarction (MI), abnormal echocardiogram, carotid intimal thickness, or abnormal ankle-brachial index have been detected in 22 percent of women and 33 percent of men aged 65 to 70 years and 43 percent of women and 45 percent of men older than age 85 years. In addition, aging is associated to increased arterial stiffness and increased pulse pressure. There is an increase in fibrinogen, coagulation factors, platelet activity, increase in the levels of plasminogen activator inhibitor, resulting in impaired fibrinolysis. Inflammatory cytokines, endothelial dysfunction potentiate the development of atherosclerosis.

3. Clinical presentation

After the age of 80, a minority of patients complain of chest pain. Symptoms like angina are less frequent, ischaemia is more likely to be silent and pain description differs from the classic substernal pressure. Symptoms may be described primarily as dyspnea, shoulder or back pain, weakness, fatigue or epigastric discomfort. Some patients describe symptoms with effort, but others may not, because of limited physical activity, mental impairment or altered manifestations of pain caused by diabetes or age changes. Symptoms may occur at rest or during mental stress. Silent ischaemia has been reported in 20 to 50 percent of patients 65 years or older. Treadmill exercise testing can provide information in patients able to exercise but the specificity is reduced because of a high prevalence of resting ST-T abnormalities on the ECG of elderly patients. Exercise results can be enhanced by the use of modified low-intensity exercise protocols. Stress echocardiography or nuclear studies are very useful in case of exercise limitation or ECG alterations. The presence of coronary calcifications is not a clear predictor of cardiac events. There is a high prevalence of hypertension, diabetes, obesity, and inactivity in the elderly and efforts in improving diet and activity levels, smoking cessation, treatment of hypertension and diabetes, are better than screening with vascular imaging studies in the asymptomatic elderly.

4. Treatment

4.1 Medical therapy

In addition to life style changes and treatment of CAD risk factors, medical therapy is the main choice of treatment in most elderly patients, however revascularization, whether percutaneous coronary intervention (PCI) or coronary artery bypass grafting (CABG) should not be neglected only because of age, and should be indicated as recommended by the guidelines. Aspirin, clopidogrel, nitrates, beta blockers, calcium antagonists, ACE inhibitors, statins and partial free fatty acid inhibitors have demonstrated benefits. Precautions must be taken regarding renal and hepatic function, hypotension and interaction with other medications.

The U.S. Preventive Service Task Force recommends low doses of aspirin as primary prevention in men age 45 to 79 years old and women age 55 to 79 years old for prevention of myocardial infarction or stroke respectively when there are risks of MI or stroke but there is insufficient information regarding aspirin in primary prevention in the very elderly. For secondary prevention, there is strong evidence for the use of aspirin, given in low doses there is less risk of bleeding.

Nitrates, beta blockers, ACE inhibitors and angiotensin receptor blockers can exacerbate hypotension or postural hypotension in the elderly. Also, B-blockers may produce central nervous system (CNS) effects and calcium channel blockers, especially the dihydropyridines, can produce edema which is more frequent in the older patient. Verapamil can exacerbate constipation. Both beta blockers and nondihydropyridine calcium channel blockers should be avoided in the presence of sick sinus node disease.

Of the two early large primary prevention trials of lipid lowering with HMG CoA reductase inhibitors, one only enrolled men up to age 64 and the other had an upper age cutoff of 73 years of age. In the ALLHAT cholesterol study, both the pravastatin and usual care groups had a substantial decrease in cholesterol levels. The 9,6 percent difference in cholesterol levels between the groups was insufficient to produce significant reductions in deaths (14,9% versus 15,3%) and produced only a small, non-significant decrease in the rates of heart attacks and strokes in the statin group relative to usual care (ALLHAT Collaborative Research Group, 2002). The Lipid Lowering Arm of the Anglo-Scandinavian Cardiac Outcomes Trial (ASCOT-LLA) tested the effects of lipid lowering in hypertensive patients up to age 79 years without increased lipids but with at least three additional CAD risk factors. ASCOT-LLA was stopped after 3.3 years because of a significant reduction in the primary end point of nonfatal MI and fatal CAD (Sever et al., 2003). Regarding secondary prevention, The Heart Protection Study demonstrated a 27% decrease in non-fatal MI and coronary death in patients older than 70 years of age. The Prospective Study of Pravastatin in the Elderly at Risk (PROSPER) a study with almost equal numbers of men and women aged 70 to 82 years who either had CAD or were at risk for cardiac events showed a significant reduction in mortality, nonfatal MI, and stroke (Shepherd et al., 2002). In summary, older patients should not be excluded from statin therapy, but caution must be taken in frail patients because of a higher risk of myopathy.

4.1.1 Considerations when prescribing medications in older patients

- Knowledge of collateral effects of cardiovascular medications, specially hypotension, bradicardia or exacerbation electrical conductance defects.
- Knowledge of non cardiac medications its effects and drug interaction with cardiovascular drugs.
- Loading doses should be reduced.
- Body surface area should be used to estimate dose (loading and maintenance).
- Estimate glomerular filtration to guide dosing of medications.
- Consider lower doses with hepatically cleared drugs.
- Time between dosages should be adjusted.
- Assess non adherence of medications.
- Assess adequate financial coverage.

4.2 Revascularization

4.2.1 Cabg vs pci

There is increased experience with both PCI and CABG in older patients. Half of all PCI and CABG procedures are performed in patients older than 65 years of age, with one third of coronary artery revascularization procedures performed in patients older than 70 years of age.
The Bypass Angioplasty Revascularization Investigation (BARI) trial of patients with multivessel disease included 39% patients between the ages of 65 and 80 (BARI Investigators, 2007). It demonstrated that this group of patients had a higher early morbidity and mortality after CABG compared with PCI but greater angina relief and fewer repeat procedures after CABG. Stroke was more common after CABG (1.7% versus 0.2%, p = 0.015). Heart failure or pulmonary edema were more common after PTCA (4.0 versus 1.3%, p = 0.011) and the 5-year survival rate was more than 80 percent for both procedures, with no difference between both treatments in non-diabetics but lower than in younger patients.
The Northern New England Cardiovascular Disease Study Group included nearly 1693 patients older than the age of 80 years who were treated for two or three vessel disease, found better in-hospital mortality and short-term survival for PCI versus CABG. For those surviving past 6 months, survival was better for patients who underwent CABG. PCI data were from bare metal stent implants, and CABG data were from on-pump procedures in more than 85 percent (Dacey et al, 2006).

Elderly patients who require PCI are more likely to have complex, multivessel disease requiring multilession interventions, than their younger counterparts. Nonfatal complications with procedures increase with age. PCI is associated with a slightly less than 1 percent risk of permanent stroke or coma, and CABG is associated with a 3 to 6 percent incidence of permanent stroke or coma in patients older than 75 years of age. Interventions on calcified plaques are associated with increased frequency of periprocedural complications, decreased procedural success rates and inadequate stent expansion and increased rates of restenosis. Tortuous and calcified vessels increase the difficulty of coronary device deployment and the risk of complications, including those with vascular access. Decreased vasodilatory response to nitroglycerin, increased plasma levels of activated coagulation factors and thrombin-antithrombin complexes are higher in older than in younger adults and platelet reactivity is also enhanced. These changes contribute to increased risk of acute thrombosis.

As stated before, the metabolism of many drugs is reduced and renal drug clearance is also compromised with increasing age. The decline in renal function affects the clearanceofanti-thrombotic drugs used in patients undergoing PCI, such as low-molecular-weight heparin and glycoprotein (GP) IIb/ IIIa receptor inhibitors, and might, in part, explain the increased risk of bleeding seen when these agents are used in the elderly. Renal protection from contrast to prevent renal failure must be taken in consideration with pre and post procedure hydration with saline solution and the use of the lower dose of isosmolar contrast.

Regarding CABG in the postoperative period, longer durations of ventilatory support, greater need for inotropic support and intraaortic balloon placement, greater incidence of atrial fibrillation, bleeding, renal failure, perioperative infarction, infection, stroke and delirium are seen in older patients compared with younger patients. The duration of disability and rehabilitation after procedures is usually longer, the risk of postoperative cognitive impairment in older patients detected with neuropsychological testing has been estimated as 25 to 50 percent after CABG. Depression is not uncommon as the need for prolonged hospitalization and home-assistance after discharge. The potential need for extended hospitalization, in-home assistance and depression after surgery should be assessed. Therefore there is an increase in mortality and morbidity especially during the first 30 days.

Risk assessment should be evaluated with the Society of Thoracic Surgeons risk model (STS score) or (EuroSCORE). Nielssen et al, in 2006 published a study that compared these two risk algorithms for CABG. Risk factors for all adult patients undergoing heart surgery at the University Hospital of Lund between 1996 and 2001 were collected prospectively at preoperative admission. The study included 4497 coronary artery bypass-only operations and the average age was 66.4 ± 9.3 years (range 31 to 90 years). In this study the EuroSCORE had a significantly better discriminatory power to predict 30-day mortality than the STS risk algorithm for patients undergoing coronary artery bypass.

The Clinical Outcomes Utilizing Revascularization and Aggressive Drug Evaluation trial (COURAGE) proved that the addition of PCI to optimum medical therapy did not reduce long-term rates of death, nonfatal MI, and hospitalization for ACS in patients with stable angina but showed that patients with severe angina who received PCI had greater improvements in angina symptoms and quality of life within the first 36 months than those who received medical therapy alone (Boden et al, *2007)*. Among the patients over the age of 65 years, a similar lack of benefit of PCI was shown (OR 1.10, 95% CI 0.83–1.46). In a subgroup analysis of 314 patients, studied with nuclear perfusion, PCI significantly reduced the rate of ischaemia in those with 10% or more of myocardium at risk. In this group, there was a lower risk of death and MI. An assessment of ischemic burden might be useful when deciding between invasive and medical management (Shaw et al, 2008).

In the trial of Invasive versus Medical Therapy in Elderly Patients (TIME), patients 85 years and older, with chronic angina who were refractory to at least two antiangina medications, were randomly assigned to an invasive strategy (PCI or CABG) or to conservative medical therapy (TIME Investigators, 2001). The analysis demonstrated a decreased severity of angina in both groups, but death, non fatal MI or hospital admission for acute coronary syndrome was 19% in the invasive group versus 49% in the conservative group. In the Alberta Project for Outcomes Assessment in Coronary Heart Disease (APPROACH), in which the health status of 21,573 patients with CAD treated with PCI, CABG surgery, or medical therapy was measured, among the 6,181 patients aged 70 years or older the improvements in health status observed with coronary revascularization was better at four years than in those patients treated medically, even in patients over 80 years of age (Graham et al, 2006).

ACC/AHA Coronary Artery Bypass Surgery and PCI Guidelines conclude that age alone should not be used as the sole criterion when considering revascularization procedures. Individualized prognostic information based on multiple clinical factors and respect for patient preference in the decision-making process has a clear role.

5. Acute coronary syndromes

About 60 percent of hospital admissions for acute myocardial infarction (AMI) occur in people older than 65 years, and account for approximately 85 percent of deaths caused by AMI. With increasing age, the gender composition of patients presenting with AMI changes from predominantly men in the middle age, to an equal number of men and women and a majority of women in patients older than 80 years of age. Mortality is higher in older women than in older men with AMI, as are adverse outcomes with thrombolytics, and glycoprotein (GP) IIb/IIIa inhibitors. As age increases, there are more patients with functional limitation, heart failure, prior coronary disease, renal insufficiency and patients with prior revascularization. Fewer older patients present with chest pain or ST elevation on ECG within 6 hours of symptom onset.

5.1 Thrombolysis

Most randomized clinical trials of thrombolysis have enrolled few patients older than 75 years of age. In a study of 14,341 of Medicare patients older than 65 years with ST elevation MI or left bundle bunch block, treated with thrombolytics there was a significant reduction of mortality at one year, but with 1.5 rate of intracranial hemorrhage. The Fibrinolytics Therapy Trialists´ found a 15% percent reduction in mortality in patients older than 65 years, and there were 34 lives saved per 1000 patients. This result was more effective than in younger patients in whom 11 lives were saved per 1000 patients. Some studies that include patients up to 75 years of age have demonstrated that fibrinolytic, antiplatelet, and antithrombin therapy is associated with a survival advantage compared with placebo that may be similar to than that seen in younger patients. The Global Utilization of Streptokinase and Tissue plasminogen activator for Ocluded coronary arteries-I (GUSTO I) found a significant absolute reduction in mortality with thrombolysis, specially with plasminogen activator in patients 65 to 85 years of age. In patients older than 85 there was a beneficial trend with streptokinase. Finally, in a registry of Swedish Hearts Intensive Care Admissions, in a group of 6,891 patients 75 years and older, fibrolytic therapy was associated with a 13% relative reduction in the composite of mortality and cerebral bleeding complications at one year. Complication of minor and major bleeding, intracranial bleeding and transfusion rates are higher in older patients compared with younger patients with all agents and some subgroups may not have an overall benefit from use of thrombolytics. Those with high risk for ICH include patients older than 75 years, women, African Americans, small size, prior stroke, systolic blood pressure >160 mm Hg. Fibrin-specific agents such as tissue plasminogen activator are also associated with increased stroke risk caused by ICH in the older than 75 year age group. Improper dosing of antiplatelet, antithrombin agents or combinations with low-molecular-weight heparins or GP IIB/IIIa inhibitors increase as well the risk of bleeding. Even with dose adjustments, however, the risk of bleeding appears increased in older patients.

5.2 Antithrombotic agents

Trial data shows that aspirin reduces mortality in patients older than 70 years and is recommended for routine administration to older patients with acute MI, although older patients have been less likely to receive aspirin than younger patients in routine clinical practice. The addition of clopidogrel to aspirin reduces major events, with similar absolute reductions in patients younger and older than 65 years. In the Clopidogrel and Metoprolol in Myocardial Infarction Trial (COMMIT), a chinese megatrial with almost 46,000 MI patients, with 11,934 patients older than 70, in which half of the patients were treated with clopidogrel and the other half with placebo, there was a 9% reduction in the composite end point of death, reinfarction and stroke without an increase in serious bleeding. It also showed a significant reduction in mortality in the patients treated with clopidogrel (COMMIT Collaborative Group, 2005). Patients were treated with 75 mg. of clopidogrel without the 300 milligrams loading dose. Low- dose of aspirin ($\leq$ 100mg.) should be used when combined with clopidogrel. Prasugrel is not recomended in patients over 75 years and there is not enough information on the safety about ticagrelor. GP IIb/IIIa inhibitors appear efficacious in older patients but in patients over age 75 years when given in combination with thrombolytics there is an increased risk of bleeding. Bleeding is about twofold greater in older patients undergoing PCI who receive GP IIb/IIIa inhibitors compared with patients who do not, with intracranial bleeding as the most common site of fatal bleeds.

Antiplatelet and antithrombin agents have narrow therapeutic windows dosing should be based on weight and renal function. Prospective observational analyses have shown that more than 40 percent of patients with acute coronary syndromes receiving unfractionated heparin, low-molecular-weight heparin, or GP IIb/IIIa inhibitors receive at least one dose in excess of guidelines. Factors associated with excess dosing were older age, female sex, renal insufficiency, low body weight, diabetes mellitus, and congestive HF. Bleeding increased relative to the degree of excess dose and to the number of agents administered in excess. Mortality is higher and length of hospital stay is longer in patients administered excess dosing and there is a close relation between bleeding and mortality. Women had twofold higher rates of major bleeding than men and are three times more likely to receive excess GP IIb/IIIa doses than men. Approximately 25 percent of the bleeding risk was attributable to excess dosing in women versus 4.4 percent in men. A randomized, controlled clinical trial for treatment of acute MI with PCI with eptifibatide administration has also reported increased bleeding resulting from lack of dose adjustment for reduced renal function (Kirtane et al, 2006). Fondaparinux and bivalirudin have shown less risk of bleeding in patients with ST-elevation MI (STEMI) and non-STEMI, including the elderly.

Primary angioplasty in experienced centers is associated with improved outcomes compared with thrombolytic strategies in elderly patients with STEMI. Even when mortality is reduced with primary PCI compared with thrombolytic therapy, in-hospital mortality of patients older than the age of 75 years is estimated to be fivefold higher than patients younger than 75 years, and 1-year mortality is 7-fold greater. Achieving revascularization within 90 minutes is less likely in older patients with delays in diagnosis and/or transport to experienced centers. Acute procedural success rates are also somewhat lower than in younger MI populations, there are increased risk of bleeding, complications including those at the access site, increased transfusion requirements and contrast-mediated renal dysfunction. However, PCI is preferred to fibrinolysis as a reperfusion option for elderly patients who experience STEMI.

The Global use of strategies to open Occluded Coronary Arteries (GUSTO) IIb trial was one of the first to report that PCI is superior to fibrinolysis among all age groups, and in particular that this strategy has the greatest benefit in the elderly, when all age groups are compared (Angioplasty Substudy Investigators, 1997). The National Registry of Myocardial

Infarction (NRMI)-2, evaluated 38,787 patients in which the treatment was performed within 12 hours of onset symptoms with either an intravenous thrombolytic agent or PCI. Of these, 10,2% were treated with streptokinase or anistreplase, 77,1% were treated with alteplase and 12,7% underwent primary PCI. In patients with STEMI who were aged 75 years, this study demonstrated that there was a lower risk of the combined end points of death and nonfatal stroke with primary PCI than with fibrinolysis, owing primarily to a higher rate of intracranial bleeding (2.5%) observed in the fibrinolysis group (Tiefenbrunn, 1998). In the Senior Primary Angioplasty in Myocardial Infarction (Senior PAMI) study, PCI was superior to thrombolytic therapy from ages 65 to 79 with no advantage of primary PCI over thrombolysis in those older than 80 years of age (Grines, 2005).In the observational setting, the Global Registry of Acute Coronary Events (GRACE) showed lower adjusted in-hospital mortality (or 0.62, 95% Ci 0.39–0.96) for primary PCI compared with fibrinolysis among 2,975 patients with STEMI who were aged ≥70 years (Mehta, et al, 2004). The Tratamiento del Infarto Agudo del Miocardio en Ancianos (TRIANA) compared primary PCI and fibrinolysis in very old patients (mean age 81). It enrolled 266 patients, 134 allocated to PCI and 132 to fibrinolysis, both groups were well balanced in baseline characteristics, and it demonstrated that recurrent ischemia was less common in PCI-treated patients (0.8 vs. 9.7%, P< 0,001). No differences were found in major bleeds. A pooled analysis with two previous reperfusion trials performed in older patients showed an advantage of PCI over fibrinolysis in reducing death, re-infarction, or stroke at 30 days (Bueno, et al, 2010**)**. Finally, in a meta-analysis of 22 randomized trials (n= 6,763) evaluating the effects of primary PCI versus fibrinolysis, de Boer et al showed a mortality reduction favoring primary PCI in all age strata, as well as reductions in the risk of repeat MI and stroke.
Regarding non STEMI, it is the most frequent manifestation of CAD and represents the largest group of patients undergoing PCI. Despite the advances in medical and interventional treatments, the mortality and morbidity remain high and equivalent to patients with STEMI after the initial month. The ultimate goals of angiography and revascularization are mainly twofold: symptom relief, and improvement of prognosis in the short and long term. Different trials have shown that an invasive strategy reduces ischaemic endpoints mainly by reducing severe recurrent ischaemia and the clinical need for revascularization. The most recent meta-analysis of 3 randomized trials with a follow up of 5 years, showed a 19 % relative reduction in non fatal MI and death. This difference was mainly driven by reduction in MI. In these trials between 12,5% to 18,8% of the patients were over 75 years old, most of them in the high risk group, in whom the invasive therapy had the greatest effect. (Fox, 2010)

6. Drug eluting versus bare metal stents

Randomized controlled trials and pooled analyses of randomized trials in which drug eluting stents (DES) and bare metal stents (BMS) have been compared demonstrate similar acute and intermediate survival and MI outcomes among nonelderly patients. Elderly patients enrolled in these trials has been small and no dedicated randomized comparison trial of DES to BMS has been performed among patients aged >65 years. In a study of 71,965 elderly patients (mean age 75 years) undergoing PCI, in those in whom DES were used, there was lower adjusted mortality (HR 0.83, 95% Ci 0.81–0.86) than contemporary controls undergoing BMS implantation. DES-treated patients were also less likely than controls to undergo revascularization procedures within 2 years after PCI and had fewer hospitalizations for MI. In an analysis of 262,700 Medicare patients (mean age 73 years) treated at 650 hospitals from 2004 to 2006, recipients of DES (83% of whom were aged over 65 years) had lower risk adjusted mortality (HR 0.75, 95% Ci 0.72–0.79) and risk of MI (HR 0.77, 95% Ci 0.72–0.81) than BMS-treated patients, but had minimal differences in rates of repeat revascularization or bleeding.

7. Our experience in chile

We performed a study randomised, retrospective comparing DES versus BMS in elderly patients 75 years and older who underwent PCI. The clinical setting was STEMI in 40 percent of patients, non STEMI in 25 percent, stable angina in 24 percent and silent ischaemia in 11 percent. The purpose of this study was to determine whether the use of DES was associated with less mortality, MI (fatal and non fatal), angina and hospitalization of cardiac causes. One hundred and forty six patients were analyzed in which DES and BMS were implanted between the years 2003 and 2007, with a median follow up of 5.2 years. Twenty nine patients were selected in the DES group and 26 in the BMS group. The groups were comparable according to age, gender, risk factors, symptoms, ejection fraction, number of vessels affected and number of stents implanted (Table 1).

CHARACTERISTICS	BMS	DES	P
Nº OF PATIENTS	26	29	
PREVIOUS MI	6	6	NS*
DIABETES	9	14	NS*
HYPERTENSION	23	20	NS*
HIGH CHOLESTEROL	14	20	NS*
AGE	79,8	79,4	NS**
MALE	15	14	NS*
TOBACCO	2	3	NS*
PREVIOUS PCI	4	9	NS*
1 VESSEL DISEASE	12	13	NS*
2 VESSELS DISEASE	5	6	NS*
3 VESSELS DISEASE	9	10	NS*
LVEF > 50%	17	16	NS*
1 VESSEL TREATED	18	20	NS*
MORE THAN 1 VESSEL TREATED	8	9	NS*

* Chi-squared ** T- Student
NS: statistically non significant LVEF: left ventricular ejection fraction

Table 1. Baseline Characteristics

Both groups were compared according to global mortality, mortality of cardiac disease, presence of angina, MI and hospitalizations because of a cardiac disease. As shown in table 2, in this group of elderly patients in which a DES was implanted there were no differences in global mortality, MI and angina when compared to the group of patients in which a BMS was implanted. However, there was statistical significant less hospitalization because of cardiac disease and a tendency to less mortality because of cardiac disease.

	BMS	DES	P
N° of patients	26 (100%)	29 (100%)	0,9767
Global Mortality	9 (34,6%)	11 (38%)	0, 8117
Mortality of Cardiac disease	7 (26,4%)	3(10%)	0,98
Angina	3 (11, 5 %)	4 (13, 7 %)	NS
MI	2 (7, 6 %)	3 (10, 3 %)	NS
Hospitalization because of cardiac disease	9 (34, 6%)	5 (17, 2%)	0,0001

Table 2. Results

8. Rehabilitation

The feasibility and improvement with intensive exercise interventions have been shown for both the frailest elderly residing in the community as well as in the nursing home. The Cardiac Rehabilitation in Advanced Age (CR-AGE) trial compared hospital-based cardiac rehabilitation with home-based cardiac rehabilitation in cognitively intact patients from ages 46 to 86 with recent MI (Marchionni et al., 2003). Similar improvement in total work capacity and health-related quality of life was seen with home-based rehabilitation compared with hospital-based rehabilitation in all age groups without improvement in the control group. The improvement, however, was somewhat smaller in the group older than age 75. Benefits decreased over time after hospital rehabilitation but were maintained with home cardiac rehabilitation. Complications were similar across groups, whereas costs were lower in the home rehabilitation group.

In summary, what to consider when approaching to the older patient with CAD:

1. Morbidity and mortality in the elderly with CAD and CAD treated medically or with revascularization increases with age, especially in patients older than age 75 years.
2. Special care must be taken regarding medications, dose, collateral effects, drug interactions and interaction with other comorbidities.
3. Clinically recognized CAD or heart failure confer the greatest risk for cardiac death and warrant aggressive secondary prevention strategies.
4. In STEMI patients
   - In hospitals where direct PCI can be performed rapidly by experienced operators, PCI has an advantage over thrombolysis.
   - In hospitals without PCI capability reperfusion therapy with thrombolytic should be considered, regarding thrombolytic drugs especially in very old patients, streptokinase should be considered.
   - Avoid combinations of GP IIb/IIIa inhibitors with thrombolytics. In case of low molecular heparins and thrombolytics, lower doses as recommended can be used.

- The use of antiplatelet and antithrombotic drugs is recommended according to the guidelines but a careful evaluation of the bleeding risk should be taken.
- For non STEMI patients the same care with antiplatelets and antithrombotic drugs must be taken and the same recommendations of the guidelines regarding invasive or conservative approach must be taken.

5. Decisions regarding medical therapy versus revascularization: PCI or CABG should be based not only on symptoms, severity of CAD, left ventricular function but in the context of other comorbidities, lifestyle, projected life span, and preferences.
6. In case of PCI the patient and family must be aware of the risks but some are less explained by the physician, especially lower success, renal failure, prolonged hospitalization and bleeding. The radial approach should be preferred in order to diminish this last complication.
7. In case of CABG prolonged hospitalization because respiratory, renal, central nervous system or infectious conditions and special home care should be emphasized.

9. Conclusion

CAD in the elderly is more severe and is accompanied by a high rate of comorbidities. There are a few trials that include a significant number of older patients, therefore there is little information on how to optimize treatment in this age group. There are age-associated pathophysiological changes as well different comorbidities. Physicians tend to be more conservative and use less aggressive therapies, although it has been proven that these patients have greater benefits with aggressive therapy but also complications are more common. The elderly with CAD are also a group that is very likely to experience improvements in clinical outcomes and functional status with revascularization. The decision on when to perform revascularization in elderly patients and how to revascularize, is difficult. More than one in five patients treated with percutaneous coronary intervention (PCI) are aged ≥75 years and the proportion of elderly individuals in the population is growing. Although a slight advantage of surgical over percutaneous revascularization might exist for elderly patients with multivessel coronary disease, surgical revascularization should remain an option for a selected population of elderly patients with few comorbidities.

10. Future directions

Increasing emphasis is being placed on preventive strategies for CAD in older patients and improving the quality of care using current therapies that were not designed for the elderly. A major limitation is the lack of understanding of the mechanisms underlying many age-related cardiovascular changes or diseases. Increased investigation at both the basic level and clinical level is necessary to identify therapies that will benefit older patients on the basis of both the pathophysiology of age-related CV disease and the frequent presence of comorbid diseases. Caring for patients near the end of their lives is different than caring for patients with longer life expectancies. Research and training will be necessary to achieve coordinated care for the older patient, and both medical and social factors must be considered to provide optimal care.

11. References

Centers for Disease Control and Prevention: MMWR Series on Public Health and Aging. MMWR 2003; 52:101-106.

U.S. Census Bureau: Income 2001 (http://www.census.gov/hhes/income). Accessed July 15, 2003.

Lakatta E, Levy D. Arterial and cardiac aging: Major shareholders in cardiovascular disease enterprises: Part II: The aging heart in health: Links to heart disease. Circulation 2003; 107:346-354.

Alexander K P, Chen A Y, Newby L K et al. Decline in GP 2b3a inhibitor overdosing with site-specific feedback in CRUSADE [abstract 3527]. Circulation 2007; 116 (Suppl. II), 798–799.

Lakatta EG. Arterial and cardiac aging: Major shareholders in cardiovascular disease enterprises: Part III: Cellular and molecular clues to heart and arterial aging. Circulation 2003; 107:490-497.

Brawnwald´s Heart Disease: a Text of Cardiovascular Medicine. Chapter 75: Cardiovascular disease in the Elderly. Pages 1923-1949.

Wilkerson W, Sane D. Aging and thrombosis. Semin Thromb Hemost 2002; 28:555-568.

Willerson J. Systemic and local inflammation in patients with unstable atherosclerotic plaques. Prog Cardiovasc Dis 2002; 44:469-478. Review.

Shlipak M, Sarnak M, Katz R et al: Cystatin C and the risk of death and cardiovascular events among elderly persons. N Engl J Med 2005; 352:2049-2060.

Mieres J, Shaw L, Arai A et al: Role of noninvasive testing in the clinical evaluation of women with suspected coronary artery disease: Consensus statement from the Cardiac Imaging Committee, Council on Clinical Cardiology, and the Cardiovascular Imaging and Intervention Committee, Council on Cardiovascular Radiology and Intervention, American Heart Association. Circulation 2005; 111:682-696.

Redberg R: Coronary artery calcium: Should we rely on this surrogate marker? (Editorial) Circulation 2006; 113:336-337.

US Preventive Services Task Force: Aspirin for the prevention of cardiovascular disease: U.S. Preventive Services Task Force recommendation statement. Ann Intern Med 2009; 150:396-404.

Antithrombotic Trialists' Collaboration. Collaborative meta- analysis of randomised trials of antiplatelet therapy for prevention of death, myocardial infarction and stroke in high risk patients. BMJ 2002; 324:71-86.

Downs J, Clearfield M, Weiss S, et al. Primary prevention of acute coronary events with lovastatin in men and women with average cholesterol levels. Results of AFCAPS/TexCAPS. JAMA 1998; 279:1615-1622.

Shepherd J, Cobbe S, Ford I et al: Prevention of coronary heart disease with pravastatin in men with hypercholesterolemia. N Engl J Med 1995; 333:1301-1307.

ALLHAT Officers and Coordinators for the ALLHAT Collaborative Research Group. Major outcomes in moderately hypercholesterolemic hypertensive patients randomized to pravastatin vs usual care: The Antihypertensive and Lipid-lowering Treatment to Prevent Heart Attack Trial (ALLHAT-LLT). JAMA 2002; 288:2998-3007.

Sever P S, Dahlöf B, Poulter NR, et al. For the ASCOT investigators. Prevention of coronary and stroke events with atorvastatin in hypertensive patients who have average or lower-than-average cholesterol concentrations, in the Anglo-Scandinavian Cardiac Outcomes Trial—Lipid-Lowering Arm (ASCOT-LLA): a multicentre randomised controlled trial Lancet 2003; 361: 1149-1158.

Heart Protection Study Collaborative Group. MRC/BHF Heart Protection Study of Cholesterol lowering with Simvastatin in 20,536 high-risk individuals: a randomized placebo-controlled trial. Lancet 2002; 360:7-22.

Shepherd J, Blauw G J, Murphy M, et al. on behalf of the PROSPER Study Group. Pravastatin in elderly individuals at risk of vascular disease (PROSPER): a randomised controlled trial. Lancet 2002; 360: 1623-1630.

Gotto AM. Statin therapy and the elderly (Editorial). Circulation. 2007; 115:681-683.

Mullany C J, Mock M B, Brooks M M et al. Effect of age in the Bypass Angioplasty Revascularization Investigation (BARI) randomized trial. Ann Thorac Surg. 1999 ;67:396-403.

BARI Investigators. The final 10-year follow-up results from the BARI randomized trial. J Am Coll Cardiol 2007; 49: 1600–1606.

Dacey L, Likosky D, Ryan T et al: Northern New England Cardiovascular Disease Study Group. Long-term survival after surgery versus percutaneus intervention in octogenarians with multivessel coronary artery disease. Ann Thorac Surg 2007; 84: 1904-1911.

Kelsey S F, Miller D P, Holubkov R et al. Results of percutaneous transluminal coronary angioplasty in patients 65 years of age (from the 1985 to 1986 National Heart, Lung, and Blood Institute's Coronary Angioplasty Registry). Am J.Cardiol 1990; 66: 1033–1038.

Rizo-Patron C, Hama N, Paulus R et al. Percutaneous transluminal coronary angioplasty in octogenarians with unstable coronary syndromes. Am J Cardiol 1990; 66:857–858.

Hsu J T, Kyo E, Chu C M et al. Impact of calcification length ratio on the intervention for chronic total occlusions. Int J Cardiol 2010 (on line, corrected proof).

Batchelor WB, Anstrom KJ, Muhlbaier LH, et al. Contemporary outcome trends in the elderly undergoing percutaneous coronary interventions: results in 7,472 octogenarians. J Am Coll Cardiol 2000; 36: 723–730.

Mari D, Mannuci PM, Coppola R, et al. Hypercoagulability in centenarians: the paradox of successful aging. Blood 1995; 85: 3144–3149.

Zahavi J, Jones N A, Leyton J et al. Enhanced *in vivo* platelet "release reaction" in old healthy individuals. Thromb Res 1980; 17:329–336.

Terres W, Weber K, Kupper W et al. Age, cardiovascular risk factors and coronary heart disease as determinants of platelet function in men. A multivariate approach. Thromb Res 1991; 62: 649–661.

Newman M F, Kirchner J, Phillips-Bute B et al: Neurological Outcome Research Group and the Cardiothoracic Anesthesiology Research Endeavors Investigators. Longitudinal assessment of neurocognitive function after coronary-artery bypass surgery. N Engl J Med 2001; 344:395-402.

Jensen B, Hughes P, Rasmussen L et al. Cognitive outcomes in elderly high-risk patients after off-pump versus conventional coronary artery bypass grafting: A randomized trial. Circulation 2006; 113: 2790-2795.

Silbert B, Scott D, Evered L et al. A comparison of the effect of high and low dose fentanyl on the incidence of postoperative cognitive dysfunction after coronary artery bypass surgery in the elderly. Anesthesiology 2006; 104:1137-1145.

Johan N, Algotsson L, Hoglund P et al. Early mortality in coronary bypass surgery: the EuroSCORE versus The Society of Thoracic Surgeons risk algorithm. Ann Thorac Surg. 2004; 77: 1235-9.

Roques F, Scott D, Evered L et al. The logistic EuroSCORE. Eur Heart J 2003; 24:882-883

Boden W, Berman D S., Navon D J et al. Optimal medical therapy with or without PCI for stable coronary disease. N Engl J Med 2007; 356: 1503–1516.

Shaw LJ, Berman D S, Maron D J et al. for the COURAGE Investigators. Optimal medical therapy with or without percutaneous coronary intervention to reduce ischemic burden: results from the Clinical Outcomes Utilizing Revascularization and Aggressive Drug Evaluation (COURAGE) trial nuclear substudy. Circulation 2008; 117: 1283–1291.

TIME Investigators. Trial of invasive versus medical therapy in elderly patients with chronic symptomatic coronary-artery disease (TIME): a randomized trial. Lancet 2001; 358: 951–957.

Graham M M, Norris C M, Galbraith P D et al. for the APPROACH Investigators. Quality of life after coronary revascularization in the elderly. Eur Heart J 2006; 27: 1690-1698.

Anderson J L, Adams, C D, Antman E M, et al. ACC/AHA 2007 guidelines for the management of patients with unstable angina/non-ST-elevation myocardial infarction: a report of the American College of Cardiology/American Heart Association Task Force on Practice Guidelines (Writing Committee to Revise the 2002 Guidelines for the Management of Patients With Unstable Angina/Non-ST-Elevation Myocardial Infarction) developed in collaboration with the American College of Emergency Physicians, the Society for Cardiovascular Angiography and Interventions, and the Society of Thoracic Surgeons endorsed by the American Association of Cardiovascular and Pulmonary Rehabilitation and the Society for Academic Emergency Medicine. J Am Coll Cardiol *2007;* 50: e1–e157.

Mehta R, Granger C, Alexander K et al: Reperfusion strategies for acute myocardial infarction in the elderly. State of the art paper. J Am Coll Cardiol 2005; 45:471-478.

Brass L M, Lichtman J H, Wang Y et al: Intracranial hemorrhage associated with thrombolytic therapy for elderly patients with acute myocardial infarction: Results from the Cooperative Cardiovascular Project. Stroke 2000; 31:1802-1811.

Berger A, Radford M, Wang Y et al: Thrombolytic therapy in older patients. J Am Coll Cardiol 2000; 36:366-374.

Indications for fibrinolytic therapy in suspected acute myocardial infarction: collaborative overview of early mortality results from all randomized trials of more than 1000 patients. Fribrinolytic Therapy Trialists´(FTT) Collaborative Group. (No authors listed). Lancet 1994; 343: 311-22.

An International Randomized Trial Comparing Four Thrombolytic Strategies for Acute Myocardial Infarction. The GUSTO Investigators N Engl J Med 1993; 329:673-682.

Stenestrand U, Wallentin L; Register of Information and Knowledge about Swedish Heart Intensive Care Admissions. Fibrinolytic therapy in patients 75 years and older with ST-segment elevation myocardial infarction: one-year follow up of a large prospective cohort. Arch Intern Med 2003; 163:965-71.

Thiemann D, Coresh J, Schulman S et al: Lack of benefit for intravenous thrombolysis in patients with myocardial infarction who are older than 75 years. Circulation 2000; 101:2239-2246.

Antiplatelet Trialists' Collaboration: Collaborative meta-analysis of randomised trials of antiplatelet therapy for prevention of death, myocardial infarction and stroke in high risk patients. BMJ 2002; 324:71-86.
Sabatine M, Cannon C, Gibson, et al: CLARITY-TIMI 28 Investigators: Addition of clopidogrel to aspirin and fibrinolytic therapy for myocardial infarction with ST-segment elevation. N Engl J Med 2005; 352:1179-1189.
COMMIT (Clopidogrel and Metoprolol in Myocardial Infarction Trial) collaborative Group: Addition of clopidogrel to aspirin in 45,852 patients with acute myocardial infarction: randomized placebo-controlled trial. Lancet 2005; 366: 1607-1621.
Jolly S, Pogue J, Haladyn K et al: Effects of aspirin dose on ischaemic events and bleeding after percutaneus coronary intervention: insight from PCI-CURE study. Eur Heart J 2009; *30*:900-907.
Horwitz P, Berlin J, Sauer W et al: Registry Committee of the Society for Cardiac Angiography Interventions. Bleeding risk of platelet glycoprotein IIb/IIIa receptor antagonists in broad-based practice (results from the Society for Cardiac Angiography and Interventions Registry). Am J Cardiol 2003; 91:803-806.
Brown DL. Deaths associated with platelet glycoprotein IIb/IIIa inhibitor treatment. Heart 2003; 89:535-537.
Braunwald E, McCabe C H, Wiviott S D, et al. Prasugrel versus clopidogrel in patients with acute coronary syndromes. N Engl J Med 2007; 357:2001-15.
Wallentin L, Becker R C, Budaj A et al. Ticagrelor versus clopidogrel in patients with acute coronary syndromes. N Engl J Med 2009;361:1045-57.
Alexander K, Chen A, Roe M et al: CRUSADE Investigators. Excess dosing of antiplatelet and antithrombin agents in the treatment of non-ST-segment elevation acute coronary syndromes. JAMA 2005; 294:3108-3116.
Alexander K, Chen A, Newby L et al: CRUSADE Investigators: Sex differences in major bleeding with glycoprotein IIb/IIIa inhibitors: Results from CRUSADE. Circulation 2006; 114:1380-1387.
Kirtane A, Piazza G, Murphy S et al: TIMI Study Group: Correlates of bleeding events among moderate- to high-risk patients undergoing percutaneous coronary intervention and treated with eptifibatide. Observations from the PROTECT-TIMI-30 Trial. J Am Coll Cardiol 2006; 47:2374-2379.
van Rees Velinga T E, Peters R S, Yusuf S et al: Efficacy and safety of fondaparinux in patients with ST-segment elevation myocardial infarction across the age spectrum. Results from the Organization for the Assesment of Strategies for Ischemic Syndromes 6 (OASIS-6) trial. Am Heart J 2010; 160:1049-1055.
Lopes R D, Alexander K P, Manoukian S V, et al. Advanced age, antithrombotic strategy, and bleeding in non-ST-segment elevation acute coronary syndromes: results from the ACUITY (Acute Catheterization and Urgent Intervention Triage Strategy) trial. Am Coll Cardiol 2009; 53: 1021–1030.
Lemesle G, De Labriolle S, Bonello L et al. Impact of bivalirudin on in-hospital bleeding and six month outcomes in octogenarians undergoing percutaneous coronary intervention. Catheter Cardiovasc Interv 2009; 74:428-435.
A clinical trial comparing primary coronary angioplasty with tissue plasminogen Activator for acute myocardial infarction. The Global Use of Strategies to Open Occluded

Coronary Arteries in Acute Coronary Syndromes (GUSTO IIb) Angioplasty Substudy Investigators. N Engl J Med 1997; 336: 1621–1628.

Tiefenbrunn A J, Chandra, N C, French, W J et al. Clinical experience with primary percutaneous transluminal coronary angioplasty compared with alteplase (recombinant tissue-type plasminogen activator) in patients with acute myocardial infarction: a report from the Second National Registry of Myocardial Infarction (NRMI-2). J Am Coll Cardiol 1998; 31: 1240–1245.

Grines C L SENIOR PAMI: a prospective randomized trial of primary angioplasty and thrombolytic therapy in elderly patients with acute myocardial infarction. Presented at the 17th Annual Transcatheter Cardiovascular Therapeutics Symposium, October 16–21, 2005.

Mehta R H, Sadiq I, Goldberg R J et al. For the GRACE Investigators. Effectiveness of primary percutaneous Coronary intervention compared with that of thrombolytic therapy in elderly patients with acute myocardial infarction. Am Heart J 2004; 147: 253–259.

Bueno H, Bertriu A, Heras M. et al. Primary angioplasty vs. fibrinolysis in very old patients with acute myocardial infarction: TRIANA (Tratamiento del Infarto Agudo de miocardio en Ancianos) Eur Heart J 2010; 32: 51-60.

de Boer S P, Westerhout C M, Simes R J et al. for the PCAT-2 Trialists Collaborators Group. Mortality and morbidity reduction by primary percutaneous coronary intervention is independent of the patient's age. JACC Cardiovasc Interv 2010; 3: 324–331.

Fox K A, Clayton T C, Damman P, et al. Long term outcome of a routine versus selective invasive strategy in patients with non ST-segment elevation acute coronary syndrome a meta-analysis of individual patient data. J Am Coll Cardiol 2010; 55: 2435-2445.

Groeneveld, P W, Matta M A., Greenhut A P et al. Drug-eluting compared with bare-metal coronary stents among elderly patients. J Am Coll Cardiol 2008; 51: 2017-2024.

Douglas P S, Brennnan J M, Anstrom K J, et al. Clinical effectiveness of coronary stents in elderly persons: results from 262,700 Medicare patients in the American College of Cardiology–National Cardiovascular Data Registry. J Am Coll Cardiol 2009; 53: 1629–1641.

Fattirolli F, Cartei A, Burgisser C, et al. Aims, design and enrollment rate of the Cardiac Rehabilitation in Advanced Age (CR-AGE) randomized, controlled trial. Aging (Milano). 1998; 5: 368-376.

6

Refractory Angina Pectoris: Focus on Cell Therapy

Giulio Pompilio, Marco Gennari, Elisa Gambini, Beatrice Bassetti and Maurizio C. Capogrossi
Centro Cardiologico Monzino IRCCS, Milan
Italy

1. Introduction

Although medical and surgical treatments often provide adequate solutions for individuals with coronary artery disease, an increasing need exists to develop treatment modalities for those patients with angina who are unresponsive to medical therapy, have serious coronary atherosclerosis, and are not eligible for percutaneous techniques or bypass surgery, a condition known as *refractory angina pectoris*.

In recent years, alternative experimental therapeutic options (e.g. ranolazine, enhanced external counter-pulsation, shock waves) have been proposed in order to alleviate symptoms and improve the quality of life in these patients.

A promising therapeutic option arising from basic research is the use of autologous cells directly inoculated into the ischemic heart. Preliminary clinical trial results are encouraging.

Aim of this chapter is to review the current knowledge on refractory angina, focusing on cell therapy from a biological and clinical standpoint.

2. Definition of refractory angina pectoris

According to the European Society of Cardiology and the American College of Cardiology/American Heart Association refractory angina pectoris is defined as:

patients with stable angina pectoris, presence of coronary artery disease (CAD) on a recently performed coronary angiogram, who despite optimal conventional anti-anginal medical therapy (beta-blockers, calcium antagonists, short- and long-acting nitrates) have severe angina, functional class 3–4 according to the Canadian Cardiovascular Society classification (CCS). In addition, the patients are not accessible for conventional revascularization procedures such as coronary artery bypass grafting (CABG) or PCI (percutaneous coronary intervention).

A strong limitation of this statement lies however on the consensus of which is the patient not suitable for revascularization. Terms such as "patients who are not candidates for conventional revascularization intervention", or even less strict descriptions such as "patients who are suboptimal candidates for angioplasty or coronary bypass surgery", have commonly been used by investigators. The lack of standardized criteria not only may generate ambiguity but also make challenging to investigate the potential impact of new treatments. There are some criteria that allow to put patients into this definition: patients who are at high risk for invasive procedures (CABG or PCI) or those who we do not expected to achieve significant and stable results for anatomical reasons, despite the recent advancements of bypass surgery (off-pump coronary by-pass surgery, total arterial revascularization, etc) and of PCI (drug eluting stents, interventional approaches to a degenerated saphenous vein graft using a wide range of distal embolic protection devices and potentially new generations of stent grafts). The keystone is probably to put particular attention on the individual patients' history and symptoms. In particular, there are two aspects that has to taken into an account: the lack of improvement after optimization of the standard medical therapy and the level of patient's discomfort (in terms of quality of life, angina chest pain, shortness of breath, etc).

DEFINITION OF REFRACTORY ANGINA PECTORIS BY THE JOINT STUDY GROUP

Refractory angina pectoris is a chronic condition characterized by the presence of angina caused by coronary insufficiency in the presence of coronary artery disease which cannot be controlled by a combination of medical therapy, angioplasty and coronary bypass surgery. The presence of reversible myocardial ischemia should be clinically established to be the cause of the symptoms. Chronic is defined as a duration of more than 3 months

3. Epidemiology

Available estimates suggest that refractory angina pectoris affects between 600,000 and 1.8 million people in the United States, with as many as 50,000 new cases each year. Approximately 30,000 to 50,000 new cases per year are also estimated in continental Europe. Canadian Community Health Survey (2000/2001) data suggest that approximately 500,000 Canadians are living with unresolved angina, but these data are limited by their reliance on self-report. The proportion of these patients living with true refractory angina is not known.
Despite wide variation in methods used to derive population estimates, there is a general consensus that the incidence and prevalence of this condition will continue to rise across countries as CAD-related survival rates continue to increase and populations age.
The European Society of Cardiology (ESC) Joint Study Group on the Treatment of Refractory Angina has stressed the critical importance of systematic evaluation of the epidemiology of refractory angina pectoris to more accurately project disease burden and related health services demands. Such data point out the high relevance of the problem related to the refractory angina pectoris in terms of economic costs and human resource that are necessary to face this disease.

4. Features and diagnosis

4.1 Anatomo-physiological basis of myocardial ischemia

The anatomo-pathological base of the refractory angina pectoris is a well-known process called *atherosclerosis*, a chronic inflammatory disease of the artery - in this specific case the coronary arteries - that causes the progressive narrowing of the epicardial (and sometimes the intramural) coronary arteries by the development of a lesion called *atheroma* or *atherosclerotic plaque* causing the discrepancy between myocardial blood flow and myocardial energetic and oxygen demand, especially during exercise. The latter situation leads to the production of a series of biochemical signals such as potassium, lactate, adenosine, bradykinin, and prostaglandins that could elicit some high threshold nerves ending in the myocardium mediating the typical symptomatology of the myocardial ischemia (i.e. fatigue, thoracic pain and shortness of breath). Recent evidences suggest that both α and β adreno-receptors are involved in the biochemical signaling of myocardial ischemia. In particular, while the β-receptor is mainly involved in the sympathetic activation during myocardial stress, the α-receptor seems to play a central role in the activation of the adaptive process. Furthermore, receptors localized on primary afferents sympathetic postganglionic neurones, and dorsal laminae of the spinal cord and of the brainstem are involved in analgesia and play a role in vasomotor control.

The role of the *vagus nerve* is still not well defined. As observed by *DeJongste & coworkers* while both vagal and sympathetic afferent fibers contribute to the increased activity of spinothalamic tract cells. Activation of vagal afferent fibers could modulate the processing of information of the thoracic spinothalamic tract cells receiving afferent input from the heart, by activating supraspinal pathways and nuclei. Abandoned the old idea that activation of vagal afferent fibers may lead to visceral pain, except in the neck and jaw regions, now we know that the vagal afferents may serve as an important rapid signaling pathway for communicating the immune changes from the periphery to the areas in the brain that respond to infection and inflammation. Depending on the integrity of the vagal afferent pathway, the release of inflammatory cytokines like interleukin (IL)-1, IL-6, IL-1b, and TNFα (tumor necrosis factor α), trigger several systemic responses. This reaction induces alterations in pain sensitivity and metabolism, hyperthermia, and increased release of adrenocorticotropin, glucocorticoids, and liver acute phase proteins. Furthermore, vagal afferent stimulation activates the hypothalamus-pituitary-adrenal axis. Finally, the activation of this vagal pathway to supraspinal structures, such as the hypothalamus and the amygdala, may activate descending antinociceptive pathways that may provide projections of a visceral organ against local inflammatory reactions.

In conclusion the vagus nerve seems to play an important role in the conduction of the pain stimulus from the periphery (i.e. ischemic myocardium) to the cortical network and in the visceral response to it mediated by different neuro-hormonal pathways.

4.2 Clinical features

There is a sort of threshold limit of ischemia that may start the typical complaints of a patient suffering from angina. This patient on exercise, or under other circumstances that can increase the oxygen demand from the myocardium (i.e. emotions, cold, smoking, etc) usually complains a characteristic thoracic pain, specifically precordial pain, or a more general thoracic discomfort (that may be constrictive, suffocating, burning) often irradiating to the left arm (ulnar side), neck, throat, jaw and upper abdomen (always above the umbilicus). This situation may be accompanied with autonomic reflexes: cold sweating, nausea, vomiting, ipotension, and in general with an automatic attempting of the patient to obtain relief from symptoms by immediately putting himself at rest e stop doing actions that was doing when the pain began.

The vagus nerve is implied in the afferent transmission to the brain (particularly to the *limbic system*) and in the efferent transmission to the visceral components. Also the sympathetic arm of the autonomous nervous system plays a role in the afferent and much more in the efferent response to ischemia, promoting the *"fight or fly"* response to stress by increasing the release of numerous stress-related hormones (epinephrine, norepinephrine,

glucocorticoid, etc). If the discomfort/pain is severe the patient may experience a terrifying sensation of "impending death" that could put him in a serious state of anxiety.
Typical pattern of a stable chronic angina in that the symptoms generally regress spontaneously at rest or by the aid of some medications in less of 20 minutes from the beginning. This is generally sufficient to not loose important quantity of myocardial tissue from the ischemic injury. *Typically, patients with refractory angina maintain a good left ventricular function.*
Generally speaking, patients with chronic refractory angina differ from the ordinary angina patient in three ways: first, patients with chronic refractory angina pectoris maintain their left ventricular function despite severe three vessel disease; second, they do not experience severe arrhythmias and therefore their mortality is only about 5%; and third, their angina is very debilitating.
Regarding quality of life, there are several considerations that a physician must take into an account. First of all, we know from the history of patients that this disease only allows limited activities, and thus his day-by-day life is severely restricted by symptoms. Secondly, the psychological impact of the angina is itself cause of stress on patient and on cure-givers. For these reasons, any attempt is welcome to improve quality of life in a patient with refractory angina. Moreover, any improvement in myocardial perfusion in these patients may have a beneficial impact on prognosis.

CLINICAL FEATURES OF CHRONIC REFRACTORY ANGINA PECTORIS
THORACIC PAIN OR DISCOMFORT ESPECIALLY ON EXERCISE
RELIEF OF SYMPTOMS BY REST AND/ OR MEDICATION (NITRATES)
SEVERAL EPISODES OF PAIN IN A DAY
SEVERELY RESTRICTED DAY-BY-DAY LIFE
NEGATIVE PSYCHOLOGICAL IMPACT TO THE PATIENT AND FAMILY
INCREASED SOCIAL COSTS FOR FREQUENT HOSPITALIZATIONS

4.3 Diagnosis

The clinical diagnosis of refractory angina pectoris is basically made on symptoms.
These patients have often a heavy clinical history of coronary artery disease, with several repeated percutaneous transluminal coronary angioplasty (PTCA) procedures or one or more operations of coronary artery bypass graft surgery (CABG).
A history of severe stable chronic angina (Canadian Functional Class 3-4) despite optimal conventional pharmacological therapy and ineligibility for conventional procedures of revascularization identify the patient with refractory angina. *Stress and rest imaging modalities (stress-echocardiography, SPECT, cardiac MR, PET) are also essential to identify location and extent of ischemia in regions of still viable muscle.*

DIAGNOSIS OF REFRACTORY ANGINA PECTORIS
HISTORY OF MYCARDIAL ISCHEMIA
PREVIUOS CABG AND / OR PTCA
EVIDENCE OF ISCHEMIA IN VIABLE MYOCARDIUM
SEVERE STABLE ANGINA PECTORIS (CCS III / IV) ALTHOUGH OPTIMAL CONVENTIONAL PHARMACOLOGYCAL THERAPY
INELIGIBILITY FOR FURTHER REVASCULARIZATION

5. Conventional medical management

The conventional pharmacological treatments for patients suffering from chronic stable angina pectoris are aimed to either reduce the oxygen demand by the myocardium and improve myocardial perfusion, all of this expecting to lead an improvement in cardiac function and relief from symptoms.

Changes in lifestyle (stop smoking, weight loss if needed and treatment of comorbidities such as diabetes, ipertension) are also warranted. Additive measures, such as lipid lowering, inhibition of platelet aggregation, and interference in the renin-angiotensin system have also become established treatments for stable angina pectoris.

5.1 Nitrates

Nitrates are the first-line option to treat angina and work to promote vasodilation, thus decreasing preload and myocardial oxygen demand. They are subject to tachyphylaxis phenomenon, so they should be discontinued for at least 8-12 hours a day (generally during the night) to maintain their therapeutic effectiveness. Side effects are hypotension, headache, metahemoglobin, stomachache. An important contraindication is cerebral ischemia; caution should be done in case of assumption of alcohol and some medications (sildenafil). Nitrates have not to be suddenly suspended (rebound effect).

They are administered by different routes of administration: sublingual, spray, IM and IV.

NITRATES
NYTROGLYCERINE, ISOSORBIDE MONONITRATE, ISOSORBIDE DINITRATE

5.2 β – Blockers

Together with nitrates are first-line choice, if no contraindications exist. By virtue of their inotrope and chronotrope negative effect they reduce the heart work and oxygen demand from myocardium. Net evidence from different clinical trials have demonstrate the improvement in the survival rate in patients with coronary artery disease treated with β-blockers agents; those patient have also decreased the relative risk to suffer from another myocardial infarction. Contraindications are severe heart failure, COPD and heart block.

Β- BLOCKERS
ATENOLOL, METOPROLOL, BISOPROLOL, CARVEDILOL

5.3 Calcium channel blockers

This category of drug cause vasodilation by blocking the calcium ions flow in the smooth muscular cells of the arteries and less of the veins. They are the first-line option in the Prinzmetal's angina caused by coronary vasospasm; they are also employed in chronic stable angina when other agents are contraindicated or ineffective. Some of these agents cause tachycardia (niphedipin) while others induce bradycardia (verapamil, diltiazem).

CALCIUM CHANNEL BLOCKERS
NIPHEDIPIN, AMLODIPIN, NICARDIPIN, VERAPAMIL, DILTIAZEM

5.4 Other medications

Antiplatelet agents are useful in the secondary prevention of myocardial infarction. Statins are employed in the treatment of dyslipidemia to reduce LDL-C serum levels and improve HDL-C ones in order to reduce the progression of the atherosclerotic plaques; they also possess antiproliferative and antioxidant properties. ACE inhibitors and ARBs (angiotensin receptor blockers) modulate the renin-angiotensin-aldosterone pathway and so they improve the left ventricular function reducing the ventricular remodeling.

OTHER AGENTS
ASPIRIN, CLOPIDOGREL, TICLOPIDINE, ROSUVASTATIN, PRAVASTATIN, SIMVASTATIN, CAPTOPRIL, RAMIPRIL, LISINOPRIL, ENALAPRIL, FOSINOPRIL, VALSARTAN, LOSARTAN, IRBESARTAN, TELMISARTAN

5.5 Ranolazine

Ranolazine, approved by the Food and Drug Administration in 2006, was the first specific novel medical therapy available for the treatment of chronic stable angina after the introduction of calcium channel blockers, in the 1980s . Ranolazine is a proven antianginal agent that, unlike beta-blockers, nitrates, or calcium channel blockers, does not affect either heart rate or blood pressure. Its mechanism of action is primarly due the ability to influence the Na+ and Ca2+ homeostasis in cardiomyocytes. In particular, ranolazine's mechanism of action primarily involves inhibition of the late Na+ flux. By this effect, ranolazine prevents intracellular calcium overload and its subsequent deleterious electrical and mechanical effects. Ranolazine attenuates the abnormally prolonged and dysfunctional myocardial contraction that increases myocardial oxygen demand and, at the same time, is thought to improve coronary blood flow and myocardial oxygen supply by optimizing diastolic function. Randomized clinical studies have been performed to test ranolazine's ability to reduce angina symptoms.

The MARISA (Monotherapy Assessment of Ranolazine in Stable Angina) investigation, a double-blind, multicenter, randomized trial in which were involved 191 patients, evaluated improvements of stress-induced angina. Exercise testing was performed at the conclusion of each treatment phase, during both peak (four hours after dosing) and trough (12 hours after dosing) plasma ranolazine concentrations, to assess the sustainability of a clinical response and establish a dose-response relationship. The MARISA investigators found that ranolazine 500 mg, 1000 mg, and 1500 mg twice daily incrementally increased exercise duration relate to the assumption of placebo. These improvements were all significant when compared with placebo. Furthermore, dose-related increases in exercise duration at peak, as well as trough, and peak times to 1 mm ST segment depression, and times to angina onset were also demonstrated ($P < 0.005$). *The use of ranolazine is recommended in patients with chronic angina in combination with standard therapy.*

6. Shock wave therapy

Cardiac shock wave therapy (CSWT) is a novel, noninvasive intervention that may ameliorate myocardial ischemia and improve cardiac function. Early clinical trials performed showed that CSWT alleviated angina symptoms and improved cardiopulmonary performances in patients with myocardial ischemia. More and more evidences indicate that CSWT may reduce the ischemic burden and provide angina relief by promoting angiogenesis and revascularization in ischemic myocardium. Earlier in vivo animal studies and human clinical studies demonstrated that low-energy pulse waves produced by CSWT induced a sort of "cavitation effect" (micron-sized violent bubble collapse within and outside cells), exerting a mechanical shear force on myocardial and vascular endothelial cells. Furthermore, improved regional myocardial blood flow and capillary density were also observed.

Clinical studies corroborated these early findings, as myocardial perfusion in ischemic regions was enhanced following CSWT. In a recent study by *Yu Wang* and colleagues good clinical outcomes are reported. Investigators described improved regional cardiac systolic function and imaging studies demonstrated increased myocardial blood flow in ischemic myocardium, supporting the notion of CSWT-mediated promotion of angiogenesis. In that study CSWT procedure was well tolerated, performed without anesthesia, and allowed for concurrent monitoring of ECG, blood pressure, and blood oxygen saturation. One important limitation of current clinical experience with CSWT is the small number of patients enrolled and the relatively short follow-up period. Further larger clinical trials are expected to more reliably evaluate the outcomes of this new approach to chronic myocardial ischemia.

7. Cell therapy in refractory ischemia

The clinical limitations of the efficiency of conventional approaches justify the search for new therapeutic options. Regenerative medicine can be considered the next step in the evolution of organ replacement therapy. It is driven largely by the same health needs as transplantation and replacement therapies, but aims further than traditional approaches (*Daar, 2007*). In fact, its purpose is not just replacing the malfunctioning organs, but providing the elements required for *in vivo* repair, to devise replacements that seamlessly integrate with the living body, and to stimulate and support the body's intrinsic capacities to regenerate and to heal itself (*Greenwood, 2006*). Tissue ischemia is a promising platform for cell-based therapies. Ideally, the induction of vascularisation into an ischemic region might decrease the lesion size, prevent loss of cells through apoptosis and might inhibit the development of organ failure.

The increasing knowledge on the role of circulating cells deriving from the bone-marrow, called endothelial progenitor cells (EPCs), on cardiovascular homeostasis in physiologic and pathologic condition, have prompted the clinical use of these cells to relieve ischemia (*Krenning, 2009*). The biological rational and the initial clinical results of the use of EPCs in refractory ischemia will be hereafter discussed.

7.1 Endothelial progenitor cells

7.1.1 Biology

The discovery of bone marrow(BM)-derived endothelial progenitor cells (EPCs) circulating in the blood vessel system by *Asahara et al.* in 1997 has resulted in a new paradigm for endothelial regeneration and introduced a potential new approach to the treatment of cardiovascular disease. EPCs are adult progenitor cells, which have the capacity to proliferate, migrate and differentiate into endothelial lineage cells but they have not yet acquired characteristics of mature endothelial cells (ECs) (*Urbich, 2004*).

These cells induce neo-vascularization through paracrine stimulation (*Yoon, 2005*) and became incorporated in the wall of newly formed vessels when injected into animal models of hind limb ischemia (mouse and rabbits). EPCs cells can be localized in the adult BM

(*Peichev, 2000*), in the peripheral blood (PB) (*Asahara, Matsumoto, 2000*) and in the human umbilical cord blood (UCB) (*Pasino, Naruse, Ma, Liew*).
In the adult life, EPCs, are supposed to derive from the hemangioblasts and can be expanded ex vivo from CD34+/CD133+/KDR+/CD45+/- cells. EPCs are distinguished in "early" and "late" based on the different timing of their appearance and differences in the clones shape (*Hur, 2004*). Yoon and colleagues demonstrated that the induction of neo-vascularization by early EPCs in vivo occurs through paracrine stimulation, while late EPCs directly contribute to formation of novel vessels. Another distinction between early and late EPCs has been established with the finding that early EPCs, also named colony forming unit-endothelial cells (CFU-ECs), originate from CD34+/CD133+/KDR+/CD45+ cells in the MNCs cellular fraction while late EPCs, also named *endothelial colony forming cells* (ECFCs) originate from CD34+/CD133-/KDR+/CD45- cells (*Timmermans, Ingram, Prater*). Other cell types present in BM and PB mononuclear fractions are considered EPCs. For example, it has been shown that CD14+ monocytes have angiogenic activity (*Pujol*) and that certain subsets of T-lymphocytes also behave as EPCs (*Asahara, Gehling*).
Stem cells that can be differentiate into EPCs exist in a quiescent state associate with bone marrow niches. In the microenvironments EPCs can either remain in an undifferentiated and quiescent state or differentiate. Under physiologic conditions only a small number of these cells are maintained in peripheral circulation, where they contribute to endothelial and vascular homeostasis. In response to vascular injury or physiological stress, EPCs can be mobilized from the BM and recruited to the damage area (Pesce). Increase of peripheral blood EPCs can be induced by a variety of signal from the periphery, including angiogenic growth factors (VEGF-A, SDF-1, G-CSF) cytokines (GM-CSF), hormones (EPO, estrogen) or drugs (statins) and home to areas of ischemic injury, where they integrate into growing vessels (*Zammaretti, 2005*). In fact, EPC levels are generally low in healthy subjects, decrease in chronic vascular disease and transiently increase during acute vascular damage (*Barsotti, 2009*).
There is evidence that patients with risk factors (diabetes, hypertension, high cholesterol, smoking, obesity and metabolic syndrome) have dysfunctional endothelial progenitors; in fact their numbers are reduced in the circulation, they have a reduced migratory activity, impaired clonogenicity and survival and, thereby, a reduced in vivo neo-vascularization capacity. Similar function alteration have been reported in EPCs isolated from aged and/or male individuals and from patients with coronary artery disease or ischemic cardiomyopathy (*Hung, 2009*).
EPC reduction may have different causes, such as an exhaustion of the pool of progenitor cells in the bone marrow, a reduced mobilization, survival or differentiation (*Barsotti, 2009*).

7.1.2 Role in ischemia

The advantage of EPCs therapeutic use depends on their ability to integrate into newly forming vessels (ECFCs) or to activate neo-vascularization by pararcine mechanisms (CFU-ECs). The two distinct, direct and indirect, ways of human EPC types participation to neo-vascularization process may represents two different modalities for biologically treating ischemic disorders at the heart or peripheral levels. In fact, while CFU-ECs have a predominantly paracrine angiogenic activity, ECFCs have a modest paracrine effect and may be thus useful for long term engrafting into ischemic tissues or promote re-endothelization of injured vessels (*Young, 2007*). The positive contribution of EPCs to adult neo-vascularization has been considered an useful approach in order to attenuate myocardial ischemia in coronary artery disease. For example, when EPCs were delivered in animal models of myocardial ischemia via either systemic administration or direct intramyocardial injection, they were found in the infarcted tissue and contributed to neo-vascularization, thereby diminishing the infarct size (*Kawamoto,2006*). An important feature of EPCs is their ability to promote rapid re-endothelialization of carotid vessels denuded as a consequence of balloon-injury (*Griese, 2003*). One of the principal mechanisms in this framework appears to be the release of vasculoprotective molecules, such as nitric oxide (NO). In particular, the endothelial-specific NO Synthase (eNOS) exerts pleiotropic cytoprotective effects in the vessel wall, reduces oxidative stress, modulates vascular tone and platelet adhesion, and impairs the development of atherosclerosis. It has been shown that EPCs overexpressing eNOS have an enhanced antiproliferative in vivo effect that significantly reduced the neointimal hyperplasia (*Kong*). A study by Werner at al showed that blood levels of CD34+ KDR+ EPCs are inversely correlated with cardiovascular events and death from cardiovascular causes. These findings implied that EPCs support the integrity of vascular endothelial cells (*Werner, 2005*). EPCs also exert a significant reduction in collagen deposition, apoptosis of cardiomyocytes and cardiac remodeling (*Itescu, 2003*). Finally, Hinkel and co-workers, showed that Embryonic EPCs (eEPCs) exert post-ischemic cardioprotection by paracrine factors activating the phosphoinositide 3-kinase (PI3K)/AKT signaling pathway in cardiomyocytes in vitro and in vivo (after ischemia and reperfusion in a preclinical pig model). eEPCs were capable of reducing the amount of adhesive inflammatory cells. In particolar they found that Tβ4, one of the most highly expressed AKT-activating factors in their eEPC population, is indeed responsible for cardiomyocyte protection.

7.2 Choice of cell type and source for clinical use

The observation that bone marrow elements contribute to cardiac repair in the ischemic heart served as the rationale for adult bone marrow cell therapy after ischemic event. This evidence that precursors of endothelial cells exist within the mononuclear cell fraction of adult bone marrow forms the basis for the use of *bone marrow mononuclear cells* (BMMNCs) in clinical trials (*Oettgen,2006*).

Many studies were in agreement that administration of autologous cells in the heart is safe, and it causes an improvement, although modest, in some clinical endpoints such as left ventricular function and clinical status.

Because the numbers of autologous EPCs from peripheral blood or cord blood are limited, a great amount of attention has been directed to autologous whole bone marrow mononuclear cells (*Zammaretti, 2005*). Several investigators have chosen to deliver unfractionated bone marrow–derived cells, a technique that has the advantage of minimizing extensive ex vivo manipulation of the cells to isolate and expand a selected population of cells (*Oettgen, 2006*). The potential disadvantage of delivering a mixture of cells is that the percentage of cells that are therapeutically useful may be small. Moreover, because whole mononuclear cell preparations contain monocytic cells, it remains to be determined whether the improvement is in part aided by the monocytic cell fraction. A concern in using whole bone marrow mononuclear cells is potential unwanted side effects such as growth of bone or fibrosis from mesenchymal and stromal stem cells contained in this population (*Zammaretti, 2005*). An alternative strategy is to isolate purer populations of cells that express specific antigens.

These was clearly demonstrated by comparing in a rat model the administration of total MNCs, $CD34^+$ cells, and a higher dose of total MNCs containing the same number of $CD34^+$ cells of the stem cell treatment group. The $CD34^+$ cell receiving group was the best in terms

of capillary density, fibrosis area, shortening fraction and echocardiographic measurements (Kawamoto). Douglas et al. showed in a randomized trial in patients with intractable angina, feasibility, safety and bioactivity of intramyocardial injection of autologous CD34+ cells. Despite this, a growing body of evidences suggests that CD133 could be a useful marker that identifies a more primitive human progenitor subpopulation compared to CD34. Moreover, in addition to haematopoiesis, $CD133^+$ cells have been shown to possess endothelial capacity (*Bhatia, 2001*). Other reports of different groups, (*Stamm et al., Pompilio et al., Losordo et al.*) showed that intramyocardial delivery of purified CD133+ cells is safe; if associated with coronary artery bypass grafting (CABG) surgery, it provides beneficial effects and if used for refractory myocardial ischemia improves heart perfusion.
Another study by Freund and coworkers directly compared $CD34^+$ and $CD133^+$ cells isolated from 10 individual healthy donors. Although they did not find differences in terms of cell expansion properties, they found a greater subpopulation of more committed cells in the $CD34^+$ group and a lower long term colony-forming units (LTC-FU). Moreover, $CD34^+$ cells contained a higher proportion of erythroid colony-forming cells, whereas the highest content of myeloid colony-forming cells were in the $CD133^+$ selected cells (*Freund, 2006*). From all these results we can conclude that CD133 could be a useful antigen to select progenitor cells for a therapeutic purpose.
Many trials focused the attention on mobilizing cells from bone marrow by different regimens of growth factors stimulation. While many cytokines have been used in preclinical models, at the clinical level only G-CSF received sufficient priority. Use of this factor in patients is facilitated by its already available clinical approval to mobilized and collect HSCs for hematologic transplantation by apheresis (*Pesce, 2011*).

7.3 Route of administration

The optimal delivery route with regard to safety and efficacy remains to be established. Three main route of cell administration of have been described: retrograde via the coronary sinus, anterograde intracoronary, intramyocardial (endocavitary/epicardial injections). In 2005, *Vicario et al* reported good outcomes with retrograde delivery catheterizing the coronary sinus via the brachial vein. However given the scarcity of clinical experiences with this technique, its role in therapeutic angiogenesis is unclear.
Intracoronary delivery (*Wang, Lasala*) is performed by the direct injection of a suspension of cells into the coronary artery of the ischemic (target) area and it is most often used after MI and reperfusion attempts rather than in a context of chronic myocardial infarction.
Direct intramyocardial (IM) injection appears to be the most promising technique due to its ability to more closely target the ischemic territory of interest and, potentially, achieve the greatest local concentration of the therapeutic solution. Preliminary experiences reported IM administration via the epicardial route under direct mini-thoracotomic surgical access after an accurate study of the electrophysiological properties of the myocardium to assess the target area of ischemic but still viable myocardial tissue (*Babin-Ebell, Van Ramshorst J, Gowdak, Briguori, Reyes, Hossne, Pompilio*).

ROUTE OF DELIVERY ADMINISTRATION OF THE CELLS
CORONARY ARTERIES (ANTEROGRADE FASHION)
CORONARY SINUS (RETROGRADE FASHION)
DIRECT INTRAMYOCARDIAL INJECTION

Subsequently, the era of percutaneous direct IM injection was advanced by the introduction of an electromechanical mapping and injection catheter using the NOGA system. This approach has the potential to be as precise as the direct surgical injection technique, while avoiding the risks of general anesthesia, surgery, and painful postoperative recovery (*Hung-Fat Tse, Beeres, Losordo*).

Concerns have been raised about arrythmogenicity of cell therapy. Available trials did not show an increased risk of developing serious ventricular rhythm disturbances related to direct injection of cells in the myocardium.

7.4 Overwiew from clinical trials

On the basis of encouraging results of preclinical studies, various clinical trials have been carried out in order to evaluate safety and efficacy of cell therapy in patients with refractory ischemic cardiomyopathy, as shown in the table below.

The clinical experience of cell therapy in a setting of refractory ischemia encompasses up to now about 250 patients, 120 involved in phase I/II and 130 in randomized controlled trials (RCTs).

Hung-Fat Tse et al. conducted the first in-human study to evaluate the safety of intra-myocardial transplantation of autologous BM-MNCs for eight patients with intractable angina. Immediately before bone marrow cell injection, NOGA system was used to perform electromechanical mapping of the left ventricle and then to guide the BM-MNCs injections to the area of ischemia. The absence of any acute procedural complications or long-term sequalae, including ventricular arrhythmia, myocardial damage, or development of intra-myocardial tumour provided a strong foundation for performing larger and more definitive trials. In most trials, EPCs were isolated from the total MNCs population via magnetic positive selection of CD34+ or CD133+ cells (Losordo, Babin-ebell, Kovacic, Pompilio, Wang). The safety, feasibility, and efficacy of intra-myocardial CD133+ cell transplantation have also been established for patients with refractory ischemia as a sole therapy in the absence of bypass surgery (Babin-Ebell, Kovacic, Pompilio).

Although the limited number of patients included in the early trials, there are evidences suggesting an improvement in therms of clinical benefits and myocardial perfusion and almost all reports has demonstrated acceptable safety profiles.

Following these reports, four randomized, multicenter trials were performed to evaluate the safety and efficacy of different type of bone marrow derived cells compared to placebo or best standard care. To our knowledge, there are no published data comparing the effect of cell therapy to specific drug for refractory angina.

Losordo et al. performed a phase I/IIa, double-blind, placebo-controlled, dose-ranging trial to evaluate the intra-myocardial transplantation of G-CSF-mobilized CD34+ cells in 24 patients with intractable angina. Patients were enrolled into 1 of 3 cohorts ($5X10^4$, $1X10^5$ and $5X10^5$ CD34+ cells/kg) versus placebo. Patient-specific procedures included G-CSF injection, leukapheresis for cell harvesting, and NOGA-mapping-guided cell injection, all of which were well tolerated with no severe adverse events reported. Favorable trends in angina frequency, nytroglicerin usage, exercise tolerance and perfusion defect were observed in patients administered CD34+ cells compared with patients who received placebo. They reported few and evenly distributed serious adverse events. Following these outcomes, a phase IIb study is under way in the United States. A recently published trial randomized (1:1) 150 patients to receive intracoronary transplantation of autologous bone marrow derived CD34+ cells. The target population included patients with class III and IV angina refractory to medical treatment and not amenable to revascularization. Serious adverse

Authors	Study design	Delivery	Cell type	Mean FU period	Safety	Results
Hung-Fat Tse et al. 2003	Phase I (8)	IM^{endo}	BM-MNCs	3 months	no AEs reported	↓ angina episodes ↑ perfusion
Vicario et al. 2005	Phase I (14)	IV	BM-derived $CD31^{+}$ cells	6 months	chest pain during procedure (x2)	↑ perfusion ↓ CCS class ↑ collateral vessels ↑ QoL
Briguori et al. 2006	Phase I (10)	IM^{epi}	BM-MNCs	1 year	acute AF 7 days after procedure (x1)	↓ CCS class ↑ LVEF ↑ QoL ↑perfusion
Losordo et al. 2007	RCT phase II (18/6)	IM^{endo}	mPB-derived $CD34^{+}$ cells	12 months	SAEs evenly distributed	↓ CCS class ↓ angina episodes
Tse et al. 2007	RCT phase II (19/9)	IM^{endo}	BM-MNCs	19 months	carcinoma of the urinary bladder (x1)	↑ exercise time ↑ LVF ↓ angina episodes

Table 1. Clinical trials of stem cell therapy in refractory angina

Authors	Study design	Delivery	Cell type	Mean FU period	Safety	Results
Babin-Ebell et al. 2008	Pilot (6)	IM^{epi}	BM-derived $CD133^{+}$ cells	6 months	no AEs reported	↓ CCS class ↑ LVEF
Gowdak et al. 2008	Phase I (8)	IM^{epi}	BM-MNCs	6 months	no AEs reported	↓ CCS class ↑ perfusion
Kovacic et al. 2008	Phase I and II (36)	IC	mPB-derived $CD133^{+}$ cells *vs* MNCs	3 months	cardiac ischemia (x4), thrombocytop enia(x2) and gout(x1)	↓ angina episodes ↑ perfusion
Pompilio et al. 2008	Pilot (5)	IM^{epi}	mPB-derived *vs* BM-derived $CD133^{+}$ cells	24 months	no AEs reported	↓ CCS class ↑ perfusion ↓ angina episodes
Jan van Ramshorst et al. 2009	RCT phase II (25/25)	IM^{epi}	BM-MNCs	3 - 6 months	pericardial effusion after procedure (x1)	↓ CCS class ↑ LVEF ↓ SSS ↑ QoL

Table 2. Clinical trials of stem cell therapy in refractory angina

Authors	Study design	Delivery	Cell type	Mean FU period	Safety	Results
Reyes et al. 2009	Phase I (14)	IM^{epi}	BM-MNCs	7 months	no AEs reported	↓ CCS class
Hossne et al. 2009	Pilot (8)	IM^{epi}	BM-MNCs	12-18 months	no AEs reported	↓ CCS class ↑ perfusion
Wang et al. 2010	RCT phase II (56/56)	IC	BM-derived $CD34^{+}$ cells	6 months	no AEs reported	↓ angina episodes ↓ CCS class ↑ perfusion
Lasala et al. 2011	Phase I (10)	IC	BM-MNCs *vs* BM-MSCs	6 months	no AEs reported	↑ LVEF ↑ perfusion ↑ QoL

FU: follow-up; IV: intra-venous; BM: bone-marrow; QoL: Quality of Life; IM^{endo}: endocavitary intra-myocardial injection; BM-MNCs: bone marrow-derive mononuclear cells; AEs: adverse events; IM^{epi}: epicardial intra-myocardial injection; LVEF: left ventricle ejection fraction; RCT: randomized controlled trial; SSS: summed stress score; AF: atrial fibrillation; LVF: left ventricular function; mPB: mobilized peripheral blood; SAEs: serious adverse events; BM-MSCs: bone marrow-derived mesenchymal stem cells.

Table 3. Clinical trials of stem cell therapy in refractory angina

events were distributed evenly between cell and placebo group. CCS class, exercise tolerance and angina frequency appear to be improved in both groups at 3 and 6 months follow-up. However, the CD34+ stem cell-treated group experienced greater reduction of sytomps. Tse et al. randomized 28 "no option" patients, class III or IV angina refractory to medical therapy to receive low-dose ($1X10^6$ cells/0.1 mL) or high dose ($2X10^6$ cells/0.1 mL) autologous bone marrow cells or placebo via a direct endomyocardial injection guided by electromechanical mapping. Compared with controls, there was a significant increase of total exercise time, left ventricle function and a lower NYHA class at 6-month follow-up, but CCS class was reduced similarly in both groups. There were no acute or long-term complications associated with bone marrow cell implantation.

More recently, a randomized, double-blind, placebo-controlled trial investigated the effect of intra-myocardial bone marrow cell injection on myocardial perfusion and LV function. The study population consisted of patients with severe angina pectoris despite optimal medical therapy and myocardial ischemia in at least 1 myocardial segment as assessed by SPECT and all patients were ineligible for conventional revascularization as determined by an independent expert. The intra-myocardial injections of $100X10^6$ autologous bone marrow-derived mononuclear cells or placebo (randomly assigned in a 1:1 ratio) were delivered after electromechanical mapping using NOGA system. In this trial, bone marrow cell injection resulted in a significant improvement in angina symptoms, quality of life, and exercise capacity, in line with precedent trials (Van Ramshots J).

The Safety and Efficacy of Autologous Endothelial Progenitor Cells CD133+ for Therapeutic Angiogenesis (PROGENITOR) trial is currently ongoing in Spain and will provide more information regarding the potential benefit of CD133+ to produce a clinically meaningful angiogenic response (see also www.clinicaltrial.com).

7.5 The road ahead of cell therapy

The current state of therapeutic angiogenesis certainly still leaves many questions unanswered. It is of paramount importance that the treatment is delivered safely. Direct IM and IC administration have demonstrated acceptable safety profiles in these early trials, and may represent a major advance over surgical thoracotomy. Once the treatment is administered, assessing the benefit remains a critical issue. Exercise testing, evaluation of angina parameters, and myocardial perfusion are routinely used to assess for bioactivity, but which most reliably endpoint reflects efficacy remains unknown.
While therapeutic angiogenesis is not ready to become part of routine therapy for refractory angina, it is crucial that we continue to learn from both encouraging and disappointing clinical and preclinical studies. The combined efforts of bench and clinical researchers will ultimately answer to the question whether cell therapy will be a suitable strategy for patients with refractory angina.

8. Conclusions

Refractory angina is still a very debilitating condition, with a negative impact on patient's prognosis and social costs. Recent advancements in pharmacological and non-pharmacological therapy open new perspectives for these patients. If promising results recently achieved by different approaches will be confirmed in the near future, it is likely that the next generation of physicians dealing with such a debilitating illness will have more effective strings in their bow.

9. References

Asahara T et al., Isolation of putative progenitor endothelial cells for angiogenesis. *Science*, 1997. 275(5302):964-7

Andréll P, Ekre O, Grip L et al,. Fatality, morbidity and quality of life in patients with refractory angina pectoris. *International Journal of Cardiology*, 2009. 147(3):377-82

Attanasio S and Schaer G, Therapeutic Angiogenesis for the Management of Refractory Angina: Current Concepts. *Cardiovascular Therapeutics*, 2010. Epub head of print

Babin-Ebell J, Sievers HH, Charitos EI et al., Transmyocardial laser revascularization combined with intramyocardial endothelial progenitor cell transplantation in patients with intractable ischemic heart disease ineligible for conventional revascularization: preliminary results in a highly selected small patient cohort. *Thorac Cardiovasc Surg*, 2008. 58(1):11-6

Barsotti MC, Di Stefano R, Spontoni P et al., Role of endothelial progenitor cell mobilization after percutaneous angioplasty procedure. *Curr Pharm Des*, 2009. 15(10):1107-22

Bhatia M, AC133 expression in human stem cells. *Leukemia*, 2001. 15(11):1685-8

Braunwald E, Personal reflections on efforts to reduce ischemic myocardial damage. *Cardiovasc Res*, 2002. 56(3):332–8

Briguori C, Reimers B, Sarais C eta al., Direct intramyocardial percutaneous delivery of autologous bone marrow in patients with refractory myocardial angina. *Am Heart J*, 2006. 151(3):674-80

Burba I, Devanna P and Pesce M, When cells become a drug. Endothelial progenitor cells for cardiovascular therapy: aims and reality. *Recent Pat Cardiovasc Drug Discov*, 2010. 5(1):1-10

Chaitman BR, Skettino SL, Parker JO et al., MARISA Investigators. Anti-ischemic effects and long-term survival during ranolazine monotherapy in patients with chronic severe angina. *J Am Coll Cardiol*, 2004. 43(8):1375–1382

Daar AS and Greenwood HL, A proposed definition of regenerative medicine. *J Tissue Eng Regen Med*, 2007. 1(3):179-84

Dejongste MJ, Tio AR and Foreman RD, Chronic therapeutically refractory angina pectoris. *Heart*, 2005. 225-230

Fernandez Pujol B, Lucibello FC, Gheling UM et al., Endothelial-like cells derived from human CD14 positive monocytes. *Differentiation*, 2000. 65(5):287-300.

Freund D, Oswald J, Feldmann S et al., Comparative analysis of proliferative potential and clonogenicity of MACS-immunomagnetic isolated $CD34^+$ and $CD133^+$ blood stem cells derived from a single donor. *Cell Prolif*, 2006. 39(4):325-32

Gehling UM, Ergun S, Schumacher U et al., In vitro differentiation of endothelial cells from AC133-positive progenitor cells. *Blood*, 2000. 95(10):3106-12

Gowdak LH, Schettert IT, Rochitte CE et al., Transmyocardial laser revascularization plus cell therapy for refractory angina. *Int J Cardiol*, 2008. 127(2): 295-7

Greenwood HL, Singer PA, Downey GP et al., Regenerative medicine and the developing world. *PLoS Med*, 2006. 3(9):e381

Griese DP, Ehsan A, Melo LG et al., Isolation and transplantation of autologous circulating endothelial cells into denuded vessels and prosthetic grafts: implications for cell-based vascular therapy. *Circulation*, 2003. 108(21):2710-5

Hinkel R, El-Aouni C, Olson T et al., Thymosin beta4 is an essential paracrine factor of embryonic endothelial progenitor cell-mediated cardioprotection. *Circulation*, 2008. 117(17):2232-40

Hossne Na, Invitti AL, Buffolo E et al., Refractory angina cell therapy (ReACT) involving autologous bone marrow cells in patients without left ventricular dysfunction: a possible role for monocytes. *Cell Transplant*, 2009. 18(12):1299-310

Hung HS, Shyu WC, Tsai CH et al,. Transplantation of endothelial progenitor cells as therapeutics for cardiovascular diseases. *Cell Transplant*. 2009;18(9):1003-12

Hur J, Yoon CH, Kim HS et al., Characterization of two types of endothelial progenitor cells and their different contributions to neovasculogenesis. *Arterioscler Thromb Vasc Biol*, 2004. 24(2):288-93

Ingram DA, Caplice NM, and Yoder MC, Unresolved questions, changing definitions, and novel paradigms for defining endothelial progenitor cells. *Blood*, 2005. 106(5):1525-31

Itescu S, Kocher AA and Schuster MD, Myocardial neovascularization by adult bone marrow-derived angioblasts: strategies for improvement of cardiomyocyte function. *Heart Fail Rev*, 2003. 8(3):253-8

Kawamoto A, Iwasaki H, Kusano K et al., CD34-positive cells exhibit increased potency and safety for therapeutic neovascularization after myocardial infarction compared with total mononuclear cells. *Circulation*, 2006. 114(20):2163-9

Kawamoto A, Tkebuchava T, Yamaguchi J et al., Intramyocardial transplantation of autologous endothelial progenitor cells for therapeutic neovascularization of myocardial ischemia. *Circulation*, 2003. 107(3):461-8

Kong D, Melo LG, Mangi AA et al., Enhanced inhibition of neointimal hyperplasia by genetically engineered endothelial progenitor cells. *Circulation*, 2004. 109(14):1769-75

Kornowski R, Fuchs S and Zafrir N, Refractory myocardial ischemic syndromes: patients' characterization and treatment goals. *Future Medicine Ltd*, 2005. 1(5):629-635

Kovacic JC, Macdonald P, Feneley MP et al., Safety and efficacy of consecutive cycles of granulocyte-colony stimulating factor, and an intracoronary CD133+ cell infusion in patients with chronic refractory ischemic heart disease: the G-CSF in angina patients with IHD to stimulate neovascularization (GAIN I) trial. *Am Heart J*, 2008. 156(5): 954-63

Krenning G, Van Luyn MJ, Harmsen MC. Endothelial progenitor cell-based neovascularization: implications for therapy. *Trends Mol Med*, 2009. 15(4):180-9

Lasala GP, Silva JA, Kusnick BA et al., Combination stem cell therapy for the treatment of medically refractory coronary ischemia: a Phase I study. *Cardiovasc Revasc Med*, 2011. 12(1):29.34

Liew A, Barry F and O'Brien T, Endothelial progenitor cells: diagnostic and therapeutic considerations. *Bioessays*, 2006. 28(3):261-70

Losordo DW, Schatz RA, White CJ et al., Intramyocardial transplantation of autologous $CD34^{+}$ stem cells for intractable angina: a phase I/IIa double-blind, randomized controlled trial. *Circulation*, 2007. 115(25):3165-72

Ma N, Ladilov Y, Moebius JM et al., Intramyocardial delivery of human $CD133^{+}$ cells in a SCID mouse cryoinjury model: Bone marrow vs. cord blood-derived cells. *Cardiovasc Res*, 2006. 71(1):158-69

Mannheimer C, Camici P, Chester MR et al., The problem of chronic refractory angina, *European Heart Journal*, 2002. 23(5):355-370

Maseri A. Chronic stable angina. In: Maseri I, ed. *Ischemic heart disease*; New York: Churchill Livingston, 1995:71–103, 477–505

Matsumoto K, Yasui K, Yamashita N et al., In vitro proliferation potential of AC133 positive cells in peripheral blood. *Stem Cells*, 2000. 18(3):196-203

McGillion M, L'Allier PL, Heather A et al., Recommendations for advancing the care of Canadians living with refractory angina pectoris: A Canadian Cardiovascular Society position statement, *Can J Cardiol*, 2009. 25(7):399-401

Menasche P. Cell-based Therapy for Heart Disease: A Clinically Oriented Perspective. *Molecular Therapy*, 2009. 17(5):758-766

Naruse K, Hamada Y, Nakashima E et al., Therapeutic neovascularization using cord blood-derived endothelial progenitor cells for diabetic neuropathy. *Diabetes*, 2005. 54(6):1823-8

Oettgen P, Boyle AJ, Schulman SP et al., Need for Optimization of Efficacy and Safety Monitoring. *Circulation*, 2006. 114(4):353-8.

Pasino M, Lanza T, Marotta F et al., Flow cytometric and functional characterization of $AC133^{+}$ cells from human umbilical cord blood. *Br J Haematol*, 2000. 108(4):793-800

Peichev M, Naiyer AJ, Pereira D et al., Expression of VEGFR-2 and AC133 by circulating human CD34(+) cells identifies a population of functional endothelial precursors. *Blood*, 2000. 95(3):952-8

Pesce M, Burba I, Gambini E et al., Endothelial and cardiac progenitors: boosting, conditioning and (re)programming for cardiovascular repair. *Pharmacol Ther,* 2011. 129(1):50-61

Pompilio G, Steinhoff G, Liebold A et al., Direct minimally invasive intramyocardial injection of bone marrow-derived AC133+ stem cells in patients with refractory ischemia: preliminary results. *Thorac Cardiovasc Surg,* 2008. 56(2):71-6

Prater DN, Case J, Ingram DA et al., Working hypothesis to redefine endothelial progenitor cells. *Leukemia,* 2007. 21(6):1141-9

Reyes G, Allen KB, Aquado B et al., Bone marrow laser revascularisation for treating refractory angina due to diffuse coronary heart disease. *Eur J Cardiothorac Surg,* 2009. 36(1):192-4

Rosen SD, Paulescu E, Frith CD et al. Central nervous pathways mediatingangina pectoris. *Lancet,* 1994. 344(8916):147–50

Sieveking DP and Martin KC, Cell therapies for therapeutic angiogenesis: back to the bench. *Vascular Medicine,* 2009. 14(2):153–166

Stamm C, Kleine HD, Choi YH et al., Intramyocardial delivery of $CD133^+$ bone marrow cells and coronary artery bypass grafting for chronic ischemic heart disease: safety and efficacy studies. J *Thorac Cardiovasc Surg,* 2007. 133(3):717-25

Sylvén C, Neurophysiological aspects of angina pectoris. *Z Kardiol, 1997.* 86(1):95–105

TenVaarwerk IA, Jessurun GA, DeJongste MJ et al., Clinical outcome of patients treated with spinal cord stimulation for therapeutically refractory angina pectoris. The working group on neurocardiology. *Heart, 1999.* 82(1):82–8

Timmermans F, Plum J, Yoder MC et al., Endothelial progenitor cells: identity defined? *J Cell Mol Med,* 2009. 13(1):87-102

Timmermans F, Van Hauwermeiren F, De Smedt M et al., Endothelial outgrowth cells are not derived from CD133+ cells or CD45+ hematopoietic precursors. *Arterioscler Thromb Vasc Biol,* 2007. 27(7):1572-9

Tse HF, Kwong YL, Chan JK et al., Angiogenesis in ischaemic myocardium by intramyocardial autologous bone marrow mononuclear cell implantation. *Lancet,* 2003. 361(9351):47-9

Tse HF, Thambar S, Kwong YL et al., Prospective randomized trial of direct endomyocardial implantation of bone marrow cells for treatment of severe coronary artery diseases (PROTECT-CAD trial). *Eur Heart J,* 2007. 28(24):2998-3005.

Urbich C and Dimmeler S, Endothelial progenitor cells: characterization and role in vascular biology. *Circ Res,* 2004. 95(4):343-53

Vadnais DV and Wenger NK, Emerging clinical role of ranolazine in the management of angina. *Therapeutics and Clinical Risk Management,* 2010. 21(6):517–530

Van Ramshorst J, Bax JJ, Beeres SL et al., Intramyocardial bone marrow cell injection for chronic myocardial ischemia: a randomized controlled trial. *JAMA,* 2009. 301(19): 1997-2004

Vicario J, Campos C, Piva J et al., (2005). One-year follow-up of transcoronary sinus administration of autologous bone marrow in patients with chronic refractory angina. *Cardiovasc Revasc Med,* 2005. 6(3):99- 107

Wang Y, Cui J, Peng W et al., Intracoronary autologous CD34+ stem cell therapy for intractable angina. *Cardiology,* 2010. 117(2):140-7

Wang Y, Guo T, Cai HY et al. Cardiac shock wave therapy reduces angina and improves myocardial function in patients with refractory coronary artery disease. *Clin. Cardiol,* 2010. 33(11):693–699

Werner N, Kosiol S, Schiegl T et al., Circulating endothelial progenitor cells and cardiovascular outcomes. *N Engl J Med,* 2005. 353(10):999-1007

Yoon CH, Hur J, Park KW et al., Synergistic neovascularization by mixed transplantation of early endothelial progenitor cells and late outgrowth endothelial cells: the role of angiogenic cytokines and matrix metalloproteinases. *Circulation,* 2005. 112(11):1618-27

Yoon YS, Wecker A, Heyd L et al., Clonally expanded novel multipotent stem cells from human bone marrow regenerate myocardium after myocardial infarction. *J Clin Invest,* 2005. 115(2):326-38

Young PP, Vaughan DE, and Hatzopoulos AK, Biologic properties of endothelial progenitor cells and their potential for cell therapy. *Prog Cardiovasc Dis,* 2007. 49(6):421-9